T0187599

Multifunctional Cosmetics

edited by

Randy Schueller and Perry Romanowski

Alberto Culver Company
Melrose Park, Illinois, U.S.A.

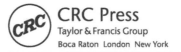

CRC Press
Taylor & Francis Group
Boca Raton London New York

CRC Press is an imprint of the
Taylor & Francis Group, an **informa** business

First published 2003 by Marcel Dekker Inc.

Published 2019 by CRC Press
Taylor & Francis Group
6000 Broken Sound Parkway NW, Suite 300
Boca Raton, FL 33487-2742

© 2003 by Taylor & Francis Group, LLC
CRC Press is an imprint of Taylor & Francis Group, an Informa business

First issued in paperback 2019

No claim to original U.S. Government works

ISBN-13: 978-0-367-44697-0 (pbk)
ISBN-13: 978-0-8247-0813-9 (hbk)

Visit the Taylor & Francis Web site at
http://www.taylorandfrancis.com

and the CRC Press Web site at
http://www.crcpress.com

COSMETIC SCIENCE AND TECHNOLOGY

Series Editor

ERIC JUNGERMANN

Jungermann Associates, Inc.
Phoenix, Arizona

1. Cosmetic and Drug Preservation: Principles and Practice, *edited by Jon J. Kabara*
2. The Cosmetic Industry: Scientific and Regulatory Foundations, *edited by Norman F. Estrin*
3. Cosmetic Product Testing: A Modern Psychophysical Approach, *Howard R. Moskowitz*
4. Cosmetic Analysis: Selective Methods and Techniques, *edited by P. Boré*
5. Cosmetic Safety: A Primer for Cosmetic Scientists, *edited by James H. Whittam*
6. Oral Hygiene Products and Practice, *Morton Pader*
7. Antiperspirants and Deodorants, *edited by Karl Laden and Carl B. Felger*
8. Clinical Safety and Efficacy Testing of Cosmetics, *edited by William C. Waggoner*
9. Methods for Cutaneous Investigation, *edited by Robert L. Rietschel and Thomas S. Spencer*
10. Sunscreens: Development, Evaluation, and Regulatory Aspects, *edited by Nicholas J. Lowe and Nadim A. Shaath*
11. Glycerine: A Key Cosmetic Ingredient, *edited by Eric Jungermann and Norman O. V. Sonntag*
12. Handbook of Cosmetic Microbiology, *Donald S. Orth*
13. Rheological Properties of Cosmetics and Toiletries, *edited by Dennis Laba*
14. Consumer Testing and Evaluation of Personal Care Products, *Howard R. Moskowitz*
15. Sunscreens: Development, Evaluation, and Regulatory Aspects. Second Edition, Revised and Expanded, *edited by Nicholas J. Lowe, Nadim A. Shaath, and Madhu A. Pathak*
16. Preservative-Free and Self-Preserving Cosmetics and Drugs: Principles and Practice, *edited by Jon J. Kabara and Donald S. Orth*
17. Hair and Hair Care, *edited by Dale H. Johnson*
18. Cosmetic Claims Substantiation, *edited by Louise B. Aust*
19. Novel Cosmetic Delivery Systems, *edited by Shlomo Magdassi and Elka Touitou*
20. Antiperspirants and Deodorants: Second Edition, Revised and Expanded, *edited by Karl Laden*
21. Conditioning Agents for Hair and Skin, *edited by Randy Schueller and Perry Romanowski*

ADDITIONAL VOLUMES IN PREPARATION

About the Series

The Cosmetic Science and Technology series was conceived to permit discussion of a broad range of current knowledge and theories of cosmetic science and technology. The series is composed of both books written by a single author and edited volumes with a number of contributors. Authorities from industry, academia, and the government participate in writing these books.

The aim of the series is to cover the many facets of cosmetic science and technology. Topics are drawn from a wide spectrum of disciplines ranging from chemistry, physics, biochemistry, and analytical and consumer evaluations to safety, efficacy, toxicity, and regulatory questions. Organic, inorganic, physical and polymer chemistry, emulsion and lipid technology, microbiology, dermatology, and toxicology all play important roles in cosmetic science.

There is little commonality in the scientific methods, processes, and formulations required for the wide variety of cosmetics and toiletries in the market. Products range from preparations for hair, oral, and skin care to lipsticks, nail polishes and extenders, deodorants, body powders and aerosols, to quasi-pharmaceutical over-the-counter products such as antiperspirants, dandruff shampoos, antimicrobial soaps, and acne and sun screen products.

Cosmetics and toiletries represent a highly diversified field involving many subsections of science and "art." Even in these days of high technology, art and intuition continue to play an important part in the development of formulations, their evaluations, selection of raw materials, and, perhaps most importantly, the successful marketing of new products. The application of more sophisticated scientific methodologies that gained steam in the 1980s has increased in such areas as claim substantiation, safety testing, product testing, and chemical analysis and has led to a better understanding of the properties of skin and hair. Molecular modeling techniques are beginning to be applied to data obtained in skin sensory studies.

Emphasis in the Cosmetic Science and Technology series is placed on reporting the current status of cosmetic technology and science and changing regulatory climates and presenting historical reviews. The series has now grown to 26 books dealing with the constantly changing technologies and trends in the cosmetic industry, including globalization. Several of the volumes have been translated into Japanese and Chinese. Contributions range from highly sophisticated and scientific treatises to primers and presentations of practical applications. Authors are encouraged to present their own concepts as well as established theories. Contributors have been asked not to shy away from fields that are in a state of transition, nor to hesitate to present detailed discussions of their own work. Altogether, we intend to develop in this series a collection of critical surveys and ideas covering diverse phases of the cosmetic industry.

The 13 chapters in *Multifunctional Cosmetics* cover multifunctional products for hair, nail, oral, and skin care, as well as products with enhanced sunscreen and antimicrobial properties. Several chapters deal with the development of claim support data, the role of packaging, and consumer research on the perception of multifunctional cosmetic products. The authors keep in mind that in the case of cosmetics, it is not only the physical effects that can be measured on the skin or hair, but also the sensory effects that have to be taken into account. Cosmetics can have a psychological and social impact that cannot be underestimated.

I want to thank all the contributors for participating in this project and particularly the editors, Perry Romanowski and Randy Schueller, for conceiving, organizing, and coordinating this book. It is the second book that they have contributed to this series and we appreciate their efforts. Special thanks are due to Sandra Beberman and Erin Nihill of the editorial and production staff at Marcel Dekker, Inc. Finally, I would like to thank my wife, Eva, without whose constant support and editorial help I would not have undertaken this project.

Eric Jungermann, Ph.D.

Preface

In the last several years our industry has seen a shift toward the widespread acceptance of, and even demand for, products that offer more than one primary benefit. A variety of technological and marketing factors have contributed to this shift. From a technological standpoint, improved raw materials and formulation techniques have improved the formulator's ability to create products that can accomplish multiple tasks. In fact, certain performance attributes that were at one time viewed as incompatible or mutually exclusive (such as simultaneous shampooing and conditioning of hair or concurrent cleansing and moisturizing of skin) are now routinely delivered by single products. From a business perspective, changing marketing tactics have also played a role in the escalation of product functionality. Marketers have become increasingly bold in their attempts to differentiate their products from those of their competitors. Thus, products that claim to have three-in-one functionality attempt to outdo those that are merely two-in-ones. For these reasons, among others, it has become important for cosmetic chemists to understand how to develop and evaluate multifunctional personal care formulations.

In this book we discuss multifunctional cosmetics from a variety of viewpoints. First, and most fundamentally, we attempt to define what constitutes a multifunctional product. The first two chapters establish the definitions and guidelines that are used throughout the book. The next several chapters describe the role of multifunctionality in key personal care categories. Three chapters are devoted to hair care, with special emphasis on one of the most influential types of multifunctional products, the two-in-one shampoo. In the last several years, two-in-ones have risen to an estimated 20% of the shampoo market, and we can trace the history and technical functionality of these formulations. Other multifunctional hair care products we explore include those designed to deliver, enhance, or prolong color as they clean or condition hair.

Chapters 5–7, 9 delve into the role of multifunctional products in skin care. After an overview of the category we discuss the growing importance of shower gels and bath products that claim to cleanse and moisturize skin in one simple step. We also address how facial care products can perform multiple functions such as cleansing, conditioning, and coloring. We then discuss how antiperspirant/deodorant products use dually functional formulas to control body odor. Chapter 7 discusses the relatively new area of cosmeceuticals—products that have both drug and pharmaceutical functionality.

While the book is primarily concerned with hair and skin care products, one chapter is devoted to oral care. There is a clear trend in this category toward products that perform more than one function; for example, toothpaste formulations have gone beyond simple cleansing by adding functionality against cavities, tartar, plaque, and gingivitis.

The next two chapters focus on specific functional categories. We discuss how to add moisturizing or conditioning functionality to products that have another primary functionality. For example, Chapter 9 deals with expanding product functionality by adding sunscreen protection; Chapter 10 describes how to include antibacterial properties in a product.

The last three chapters describe some of the executional details one should be aware of when creating multifunctional products. We discuss general considerations related to formulation and how to design and implement tests for supporting claims. We also cover legal considerations, particularly with respect to OTC monographs, in which covering more than one function can lead to problems. The final chapter is devoted to the role of packaging in multifunctional products.

Randy Schueller
Perry Romanowski

Contents

Contributors

Francis Busch   Founder, ProStrong, Inc., Oakville, Connecticut, U.S.A.

Damon M. Dalrymple   Senior Research Scientist, New Product Development, ABITEC Corporation, Columbus, Ohio, U.S.A.

Jeffrey Easley   Senior Technology Transfer Specialist, Product Development, Stepan Company, Northfield, Illinois, U.S.A.

Wilma Gorman   Senior Technology Transfer Specialist, Stepan Company, Northfield, Illinois, U.S.A.

Uta Kortemeier   Degussa Care Chemicals, Essen, Germany

Monika Mendoza   Stepan Company, Northfield, Illinois, U.S.A.

Billie L. Radd   President, BLR Consulting Services, Naperville, Illinois, U.S.A.

Lawrence A. Rheins   Founder, Executive Vice President, DermTech International, San Diego, California, U.S.A.

Perry Romanowski Project Leader, Research and Development, Alberto Culver, Melrose Park, Illinois, U.S.A.

Craig R. Sawicki Executive Vice President, Design and Development, Tricor-Braun, Clarendon Hills, Illinois, U.S.A.

Randy Schueller Manager, Global Hair Care, Research and Development, Alberto Culver, Melrose Park, Illinois, U.S.A.

Joseph W. Stanfield Founder and President, Suncare Research Laboratories, LLC, Memphis, Tennessee, U.S.A.

M. J. Tenerelli Writer and Editor, Upland Editorial, East Northport, New York, U.S.A.

Ann B. Toomey Goldschmidt, Dublin, Ohio, U.S.A.

Mort Westman President, Westman Associates, Inc., Oak Brook, Illinois, U.S.A.

Shira P. White President, The SPWI Group, New York, New York, U.S.A.

Johann W. Wiechers Principal Scientist and Skin Research and Development Manager, Skin Research and Development, Uniqema, Gouda, The Netherlands

Michael Wong* Clairol, Inc., Stamford, Connecticut, U.S.A.

---

* Retired.

1

Definition and Principles of Multifunctional Cosmetics

Perry Romanowski and Randy Schueller
Alberto Culver, Melrose Park, Illinois, U.S.A.

A popular late-night comedy television program once made a joke about a product that was a combination floor wax and dessert topping. While this is a humorous example, it does support the central point of this book: consumers love products that can do more than one thing. This is a critical principle that formulating chemists should learn to exploit when designing new products and when seeking new claims for existing products. If formulators can create products that excite the consumer by performing more than one function, these products are more likely to succeed in the marketplace. In fact, in many cases, creating products with more than one function is no longer a luxury, it is a necessity that is mandated by consumers.

This book is written to share with the reader some approaches for formulating and evaluating multifunctional products. But first, to provide a conceptual framework for our discussion, we must state what the term "multifunctionality" means in the context of personal care products. The opening section of this chapter define the term by describing four different dimensions of multifunctionality. We then discuss three key reasons why this trend is so important to this industry. On the basis of this conceptual foundation, the remainder of the chapter provides an overview of the specific product categories discussed throughout the book.

While the reader may have an intuitive sense of what multifunctionality is, there is no single, universally accepted definition. Therefore, we begin by attempting to develop a few standard definitions. We hope to better define the concept by discussing four different dimensions of multifunctionality: performance-oriented multifunctionality, ingredient-based multifunctionality, situational multifunctionality, and claims-driven multifunctionality.

1   PERFORMANCE-ORIENTED MULTIFUNCTIONALITY

Multifunctionality based on performance is probably the type that first comes to mind. Products employing this type of multifunctionality are unequivocally designed to perform two separate functions. One of the most obvious examples of this kind of multifunctionality is the self-proclaimed two-in-one shampoo that is intended to simultaneously cleanse and condition hair. This type of formulation was pioneered by Proctor & Gamble with Pert Plus in the late 1970s. Pert contains ammonium lauryl sulfate as the primary cleansing agent, along with silicone fluid and cationic polymers as the conditioning ingredients. Proctor & Gamble researchers found a way to combine these materials in a way that allows concurrent washing and conditioning of the hair. The result is a product that is able to offer consumers the legitimate benefit of saving time in the shower because it eliminates the need for a separate conditioner. Thus Pert has become a classic example of a multifunctional personal care product.

In a somewhat different context, antiperspirant/deodorants (APDs) also exhibit multifunctional performance. To appreciate this example, the reader must understand that "antiperspirant/deodorants" are very different from "deodorants." Deodorants are designed solely to reduce body odor through use of fragrance that masks body odor and antibacterial agents that control the growth of odor-causing microbes. Because they are designed to reduce odor only, deodorant are monofunctional products. Antiperspirants, on the other hand, contain active ingredients (various aluminum salts) that physiologically interact with the body to reduce the amount of perspiration produced. Because these aluminum compounds also help control bacterial growth, antiperspirants are truly multifunctional: they control body odor and reduce wetness. In this context, it is interesting to note that all antiperspirants are deodorants but not all deodorants are antiperspirants. We also point out that since these aluminum salts are responsible both product functions, they could be considered multifunctional ingredients—this type of multifunctionality is discussed later in the chapter.

This principle of performance-oriented multifunctionality has been applied to almost every class of cosmetic product. For example, the number of makeup products that make therapeutic claims is increasing. One trade journal, *Global Cosmetics Industry,* noted three cosmetic products that combine the benefit of a foundation makeup with a secondary benefit. Avon's Beyond Color Vertical Lifting Foundation is also said to be effective against sagging facial skin, Clinique claims that The City Cover Compact Concealer also protects skin from sun damage, and Elizabeth Arden's Flawless Finish Hydro Light Foundation adds ceramides, sunscreen, and an α-hydroxy acid (AHA) to smooth and protect skin. *Global Cosmetics Industry* anticipates that the combination of multifunctional claims, combined with strong brand names and affordable prices, will allow such products to thrive in the coming years. A number of other examples are cited in Tables 1–8.

TABLE 1   Multifunctional Hair Care Products and Manufacturers' Claims

Pert Plus Shampoo and Conditioner
   Provides a light level of conditioning
   Gently cleanses the hair
L'Oréal Colorvive Conditioner
   Up to 45% more color protection
   Keeps color truer, hair healthier
   Conditions without dulling or weighing hair down
Ultra Swim Shampoo Plus
   Effectively removes chlorine and chlorine odor
   With rich moisturizing conditioners
Jheri Redding Flexible Hold Hair Spray
   Holds any hair style in place flexibly
   Leaves hair so healthy it shines

TABLE 2   Multifunctional Soaps and Bath Products and Manufacturers' Claims

Dove Nutrium
   Restores and nourishes
   Dual formula
   Skin-nourishing body wash
   Goes beyond cleansing and moisturizing to restore and nourish
FaBody Wash
   Moisturizers that feed the body and exotic fragrances that fuel the senses
   Nourishes the skin
   Cleans without drying
Dial Anti bacterial Hand Sanitizier
   Contains moisturizers
   Kills some germs

TABLE 3 Multifunctional Skin Care Products and Manufacturers' Claims

Body @ Best All of You Gel Lotion
  White lotion and clear red glitter
  To moisturize and give a hint of glitter
Biore Facial Cleansing Cloth
  Cleanses
  Exfoliates
Noxema Skin Cleanser
  Cleanses
  Moisturizes
Nair Three-in-One cream
  Depiliates
  Exfoliates
  Moisturizes

TABLE 4 Multifunctional Makeup Products and Manufacturers' Claims

L'Oréal Hydra Perfect Concealer
  Foundation makeup
  Protects and hydrates with a sun-protection factor (SPF) factor of 12
Revlon Age-Defying All-Day Lifting Foundation
  Helps visibly lift fine lines away
  Skin looks smoother and softer
  Ultraviolet protection helps prevent new lines from forming
L'Oréal Color Riche Luminous Lipstick
  Rich color with lasting shine
  Moisturizes for hours, enriched with vitamin E
  Hydrating lip color
Almay Three-in-One Color Stick
  Accents lips, cheeks, and eyes in a few quick strokes
  The perfect tool that does it all
  Moisturizing color glides on smoothly
Neutrogena Skin Clearing Makeup
  Actually clears blemishes
  Controls shine and is a foundation makeup

TABLE 5 Multifunctional AntiPerspirant/Deodorant Products
and Manufacturers' Claims

Mitchum Super Sport Clear Gel Antiperspirant and Deodorant
  Antibacterial odor protection
  Clinically proven to provide maximum protection against wetness
Arrid XX Antiperspirant Gel
  Antibacterial formula works to help kill germs
  Advanced wetness protection

TABLE 6 Multifunctional Nail Care Products and Manufacturers' Claims

Sally Hanson Hard As Nails
  Helps prevent chipping splitting and breaking
  Enhances color
  Restructurizing strengthens and grows nails
  Moisturizing protection and ultrahardening formula
Sally Hanson Double-Duty Strengthening Base and Topcoat
  All-in-one moisturizing basecoat
  Protective shiny topcoat

TABLE 7 Multifunctional Oral Care Products and Manufacturers' Claims

Colgate Total
  Helps prevent
  Cavities
  Gingivitis
  Plaque
Crest Multi-Care
  Fights cavities
  Protects against cavities
  Fights tartar buildup
  Leaves breath feeling refreshed
Aqua-Fresh Triple Protection
  Cavity protection
  Tartar control
  Breath freshening
Arm & Hammer's Dental Care Baking Soda Gum
  Whitens teeth
  Freshens breath
  Reduces plaque by 25%
Listerine antiseptic mouthwash
  Kills germs that cause
    Bad breath
    Plaque
    Gingivitis
Polydent Double-Action Denture Cleanser
  Cleans tough stains
  Controls denture odor
  Keeps user feeling clean all day

TABLE 8   Miscellaneous Multifunctional Products and Manufacturers'
Claims

Coppertone Bug Sun
  Sunscreen with insect repellent
  Offers convenient dual protection in one bottle for total outdoor skin
  protection
  Protects from harmful UV rays while it also repels mosquitoes
  and other pests
  Moisturizes
Allergans Complete Comfort Plus Multi purpose Contact Solution
  Cleans and rinses
  Disinfects
  Unique package stores lens
Quinsana Plus Antifungal Powder
  Cures athlete's foot and jock itch
  Absorbing powder helps keep skin dry
Mexana Medicated Powder
  Antiseptic
  Protectant
Gold Bond Medicated Lotion
  Moisturizes dry skin
  Relieves itch
  Soothes and protects
Pampers Rash Guard Diapers
  Absorbs moisture
  Clinically proven to help protect against diaper rash

---

2   INGREDIENT-BASED MULTIFUNCTIONALITY

There is a second class of multifunctionality that does not require a product to perform multiple tasks. Even though a product is monofunctional, it may contain ingredients that perform more than one function. There are many examples of this type of multifunctionality. Consider that certain fragrance ingredients also have preservative properties. And conversely, phenoxyethanol, chiefly used for its preservative properties, also imparts a rose odor to products. To a certain extent many, if not most, cosmetic ingredients are "accidentally" multifunctional. For example, the ingredients used in skin lotions to emulsify the oil phase components (fatty alcohols such as cetyl and stearyl alcohol) also serve to thicken the product. In fact, some of these ingredients have emolliency properties as well. Therefore, in this example, a single ingredient could serve three functions in a given product. Likewise in a detergent system, the surfactants that provide foaming properties also thicken the product. While ingredient-based multifunctionality may seem trivial, it can provide a way to leverage new claims by using an existing formula.

In addition, using multifunctional ingredients allows formulators to prepare products more efficiently and economically. This approach is useful when one is formulating "natural" products that have fewer "chemicals." Since many consumers think that a long ingredient list means that the product has too many harsh chemicals, using fewer ingredients that perform multiple functions may help make the product more appealing to the consumer. In addition, products formulated with fewer ingredients may be less expensive and easier to manufacture.

3 SITUATIONAL MULTIFUNCTIONALITY

Another dimension of multifunctionality is exemplified by products that claim to be functional in multiple situations. For example, consider a product whose primary function is to fight skin fungus. Yet, such a product may claim to cure both athlete's foot and jock itch. The function is the same (both maladies are caused by a fungus), but the situation of use is different, thus essentially making the product multifunctional.

In addition to the situational uses explicitly described by marketers, consumers tend to find alternate uses for products on their own. At least one published study [1] has indicated that consumers find multiple uses for products for three primary reasons: convenience, effectiveness, and cost. Savvy marketers have learned to exploit such alternate situational uses to help differentiate their products in the marketplace. An understanding of situational multifunctionality can help support advertising that promotes new uses for old brands. Wansink and Gilmore found that in some cases, it may be less expensive to increase the usage frequency of current users than to convert new users in a mature market [2]. Defining multifunctional benefits for a product can help revitalize mature brands, and there are numerous examples of brands that have energized their sales by advertising new usage situations. For example, Arm & Hammer Baking Soda was once primarily known for use in baking. But sales dropped as people began using more prepackaged baked goods. Church & Dwight responded by marketing the brand as a deodorizer for refrigerators, and sales skyrocketed. More recently the manufacturer has also promoted the use of baking soda in products such as toothpastes and antiperspirants in an attempt to make more compelling deodorization claims for these products.

It is interesting to note that consumers tend not to stray across certain usage lines when using products in alternate situations. They are not likely to use a household product for cosmetic purposes and vice versa. Wansink and Ray [2], who explain consumers' tendency to use products in similar contexts (i.e., foods as foods and cleaners as cleaners) from a psychological standpoint, say there are mental barriers that consumers are hesitant to cross, particularly for products used in or on their bodies, such as foods and beauty products. Consumers do not like to think that the Vaseline Petroleum Jelly they use to remove makeup can also work as a lubricatant for door hinges. Cosmetic scientists must be aware of these mental barriers when attempting to exploit situational multifunctionality.

4   CLAIMS-DRIVEN MULTIFUNCTIONALITY

Sometimes marketers simply list multiple, exploitable benefits of a product. For example, a shampoo is primarily designed to cleanse hair but it also leaves hair smelling fresh and *sexy?* While this secondary benefit may seem trivial to the formulator, it may be an important fact that the marketer can choose to exploit. Such "trivial" benefits can make good label copy claims, and we urge the reader to consider these secondary product benefits when helping marketing to develop claims.

Similarly, copy writers may dissect a single performance benefit to make it sound more impressive. For example, advertising claims that describe a product's ability to soften and smooth hair, and make it more manageable, are essentially referring to the single technical benefit of conditioning. While this distinction might seem unimportant to the formulator, it is of paramount importance to marketers because it allows them to differentiate their product from the competition. Formulators should strive to leverage their knowledge of formula characteristics and look for "hidden" claims that may be useful in marketing. Chemists need to recognize that it is not necessary to base every claim to multifunctionality on quantifiable performance differences.

5   WHY MULTIFUNCTIONALITY IS SO POPULAR

5.1   Increasing Consumer Expectations

In the opinion of the authors, multifunctional products are becoming increasingly popular for three key reasons: increasing consumer expectations, maturing cosmetic technology, and expanding marketing demands. The first reason is related to consumers' desire for products that can perform more than one function; people are demanding more performance from products of all types. This trend can be seen in many product categories beyond personal care: sport–utility vehicles are cars that also behave like trucks; computers are not just calculating devices but are also entertainment centers that play CDs and DVDs; telephones are not just for verbal communication, they are capable of scanning and faxing documents. Today even a simple stick of chewing gum is expected to perform like a cavity-fighting sword of dental hygiene. The same set of growing expectations has affected the market for personal care products as well. While shampoos were once expected to simply cleanse hair, the simultaneous delivery of conditioning or color protection benefits as well is anticipated in many cases.

5.2 Maturing Technology

A second factor driving the rise of multifunctional personal care products has to do with the level of maturity of the technology used to create cosmetics. As cosmetic science has matured, it has become increasingly difficult for formulators to improve upon any single aspect of a product's performance. Consider cleansing products like shampoos or soap bars. For centuries, all these products were based on soaps, which are saponified fatty acids. Because of their surfactant nature, soaps are able to remove dirt and grease from a variety of surfaces. However, soaps also tend to dry the skin and can combine with hard water ions to form insoluble deposits, resulting in the notorious "bathtub ring." During the 1940s, advances in organic chemistry led to synthetic detergents such as sodium lauryl sulfate and α-olefin sulfonates, which were vastly superior in performance to soap. Today, the majority of cleansing products (including some bar soaps) use synthetic detergents. Surfactant technology has continued to evolve over the last 50 years, yet the same compounds created in the 1940s are still widely used because they are still highly functional and economical.

Surfactant technology has become so sophisticated that most improvements are incremental: synthesis chemists may succeed in making new molecules that are somewhat milder or that are more easier to manufacture, but it is very difficult to produce new raw materials that provide dramatically improved performance that is perceivable by the consumer. Of course, this is not meant to say that there have been no new ingredient-based technological breakthroughs in the last five decades; chemists continue to create new polymers that are more effective conditioning agents and film formers. But for many product categories, it can be difficult for formulators to make "quantum leaps" in improving the basic performance of their products because the raw materials they are using are already highly effective and cost-efficient. To create new products that demonstrate additional consumer-perceivable benefits, formulators attempt to add additional functionality to their products. Instead of concentrating on "better" cleaning, formulators have began to add secondary properties, such as conditioning and moisturizing.

By combining more than one function into a single product, formulators can satisfy growing consumer expectations. In fact, certain performance attributes that were at one time viewed as incompatible or mutually exclusive (such as simultaneous shampooing and conditioning of hair or concurrent cleansing and moisturizing of skin) can now be combined in single products.

5.3 Expanding Marketing Demands

The third reason for increasing multifunctionality comes from the business sector: marketers have become increasingly bold in their attempts to differentiate their products from their competitors'. To increase consumer appeal in this competitive age, marketers claim that their products will save consumers time by performing more than one duty at once. This strategy requires marketers to add multiple functions to their products. Thus, products that claim to have "three-in-one" functionality attempt to outdo those that are merely "two-in-ones."

The impact of these three factors has made it very important for formulators to look for ways to diversity the functionality of their products. Indeed, formulators who stay competitive in the market place are constantly striving to satisfy these diverse consumer expectations.

BOOK LAYOUT

This book was designed to examine how the concept of multifunctionality affects product development. It was compiled with the cosmetic formulator in mind and is intended to provide practical information that can help guide formulation efforts.

The first part of this book is dedicated to specific formulation issues encountered during attempt to develop multifunctional products. To this end, Chapter 2 discusses the technical challenges related to formulating products with functions that once had seemed to be mutually exclusive, such as simultaneous cleansing and moisturizing. The role of consumer and marketer expectations is examined, and a process for formulating multifunctional products is advanced.

The next two chapters look specifically at the formulation of multifunctional hair care products. Chapter 3 reviews the historical development of these hair care products. It also provides a comprehensive look at the different ingredients that can be used to create multifunctional effects in hair care products. Chapter 4 discusses the development of two-in-one shampoos, the most common type of multifunctional hair care product. This product type is particularly important because it arguably represents the most significant technical advance in shampoo technology since the development of synthetic detergents.

Chapters 5 and 6 discuss the formulation of multifunctional products for skin care. Chapter 5 provides a detailed look at the development of ingredient mixtures for multifunctionality in skin care products. Methods for choosing appropriate materials and evaluating their effectiveness for various functionalities are given. Similarly, Chapter 6 discusses formulation of multifunctional nail care products and methods for their evaluation.

Chapter 7 surveys the topic of introducing therapeutic functionalities with cosmetic products. It discusses the controversial concept of cosmeceuticals, with its associated technical and legal challenges. The chapter provides a review of some of the regulatory aspects of formulating these products and formulation considerations. Numerous therapeutic ingredients are discussed, as are methods for their inclusion in a formula. Chapter 8 examines the development of multifunctional oral care products. The various multiple functions these products can have are considered, and methods for their formulation are discussed.

The next two chapters examine specific product functionalities and how these can be introduced into numerous products. Chapter 9 looks at methods for blocking the damaging effects of sunlight. It reviews the state of technology today and suggests paths for future research. Methods for incorporating sunscreen ingredients in various formulation types are also introduced. Likewise, Chapter 10 discusses methods for adding antibacterial functionalities to cosmetic products. Specific ingredients are reviewed, as are future trends in this area of technology.

The final three chapters are related to areas that affect the development of multifunctional products but do not specifically deal with formulating. Chapter 11 reviews the techniques involved in developing claims support for multifunctional products. Numerous methods are proposed for both skin care and hair care products. Additionally, an overall strategic approach is proposed for specifically dealing with products of these types. Chapter 12 examines the role of packaging in the development of multifunctional products. Numerous aspects of the package are reviewed, along with their impacts on the functionality of the cosmetic product. The book ends with a chapter on consumer research and how it can be used to aid in the development of multifunctional products. Ideas about which product functionalities should be combined and methods for gathering this information are discussed.

The field of cosmetic chemistry is an evolving one, with products being designed to have greater and greater functionality. It is hoped that this work will provide a solid basis for all who desire to combine cosmetic functionailites and inspire the development of superior formulations.

REFERENCES

1. SB Desai. Tapping into "mystery" product uses can be secret of your success. *Marketing News,* October 22, 1992.
2. B Wansink, J Gilmore. New uses that revitalize old brands. *J Advert Res* 39 (March 1999), 90.
3. B Kanner. Products with double lives—On Madison Avenue. *New York Mag,* November 30, 1992.
4. B Wansink. Expansion advertising. In: John Phillip Jones, ed. *Advertising: An Encyclopedia.* Beverly Hills, CA: Sage, 1998.
5. Functional cosmetics: A synergy of hot trends. *Global Cosmet Ind* March 1999, p 88.

2

Factors to Consider When Designing Formulations with Multiple Functionality

Mort Westman

Westman Associates, Inc., Oak Brook, Illinois, U.S.A.

1 INTRODUCTION

From two-in-one shampoos and moisturizing facial cleansers to more exotic products such as exfoliating lipsticks and UV-protective hair sprays, multifunctional formulations have become extremely common in the marketplace. Such multifunctionality satisfies the consumer's need for convenience and the marketer's need for an exploitable product advantage. It also provides the chemist with formidable technical challenges. Overcoming these challenges will, however, require increasingly sophisticated solutions, given the intense focus that these products have received during past years.

The development of truly multifunctional products may be accompanied by significant, and at times paradoxical, hazards. Indeed, commercial success may be impaired by the very same functional properties that provide the product's reason for being. For example, the product's name alone may generate consumer concerns of overfunctionality. It is not uncommon for a moisturizing skin cleanser to be received with fears that the user (and his or her clothing) will be left with an oily film. Similarly, two-in-one shampoos are commonly received with concerns of oily buildup. Clearly, a balance in label claims and functionality must be

13

reached. Ideally, the consumer should also be provided with a means to alleviate such fears (e.g., via the availability of multiple product versions, for dry, normal, and oily skin or hair). In all likelihood, the consumers' greatest concern with these products is their inability to control the relative performance of each functionality—the fear of receiving too much of a good thing. One hopes that the product development team will learn of such obstacles and ascertain how they may be overcome through diligent consumer studies and regional market testing, not after full-scale commercialization.

1.1 Defining Multifunctionality

While the phrases "multifunctional product" and "multifunctional formulation" are commonly used interchangeably, the latter more accurately reflects the focus of this chapter, and this book, in that it unmistakably refers to a single formulation that provides more than one performance benefit. This distinction is drawn because the term "multifunctional *product*" could describe a series of conventional (single-function) formulations that are packaged in individual containers within a single unit (or kit) intended to be applied separately and consecutively. For example, many "conditioning permanent wave" and "conditioning hair coloring" kits and products contain a separate hair conditioner that is to be applied after completion of the primary (permanent wave or hair coloring) process. To qualify as a multifunctional formulation, the primary (permanent wave or hair coloring) formulation should provide a highly discernible level of hair conditioning without the use of an additional component. At times, however components of a multifunctional formulation must, for reasons of chemistry, be kept apart prior to usage. Since these components are subunits of a single formulation and are not intended to be used separately, they are considered, jointly, to comprise a multifunctional formulation.

Since most conventional formulations tacitly provide more than one benefit, the question remains: At what point should a formulation be considered to be multifunctional? For example, one would not consider formulating a general-purpose shave cream that did not leave the skin supple, a general-purpose shampoo that did not leave hair reasonably easy to comb, a facial cleanser that did not provide some degree of emollience, a hair-setting product that did not ease wet comb and fly-away, or a liquid makeup that did not leave the skin feeling smooth. Given this routine requirement, at what point should the formula be considered to be multifunctional? When the secondary functionality is particularly efficacious? When special technology is required to gain compatibility, stability or functionality? When a nontraditional combination of functionalities is involved?

In an attempt to provide a more definitive point of delineation, the following discussion will consider multifunctional formulations as providing an additional functionality of a type or level not normally expected of its primary product category. With respect to the first condition, *type,* it is becoming increasingly common for cosmetic formulations to also include a drug, or quasi-drug, treatment (e.g., antibacterial soaps and liquid cleansers, UV-protectant moisturizing lotions, pigmented cosmetics, and hair styling/holding products). Special considerations related to the formulation and testing of such drug-containing products are briefly touched upon later in this chapter but are thoroughly discussed in the chapters pertaining to the addition of sun protectant and antibacterial functionality to personal care products.

With respect to the *level* of the secondary functionality required to warrant a formulation being identified as multifunctional, it is worthwhile to note the impact of shampoos containing suspended silicone on the category of conditioning shampoos. While conditioning shampoos were available for many years, the level of conditioning imparted by these silicone-containing shampoos was far enough above that previously available to warrant the creation of a new category of shampoo, two-in-one [1]. Perhaps justifiably, owing to the immense improvement they represent, chemists and marketing personnel alike continue to treat these shampoos as belonging to an entirely different category of products instead of as evolutionary members of what was an ongoing category, conditioning shampoos. It is worthwhile to note that in a development more representative of marketing avarice than technological innovation, these two-in-ones quickly proliferated into hair and skin care products labeled as three-, four-, and even five-in-ones.

1.2 Consumer Considerations

Perhaps the most important factor to consider prior to developing a multifunctional formulation is that these products are not for everyone. More importantly, they may not be preferred by your targeted audience. It may be possible, through compelling marketing and advertising, to address the reasons that lead some individuals and demographic groups to prefer conventional products, and to resist the lure of multi functionality (Table 1). For some, however, rejection of multifunc-

---

TABLE 1 Key Reasons for Consumer Preference of Conventional Products

1. **Control of the level of each functionality.** Inability to control the level/ratio of each functionality in multifunctional products has resulted in too much of a good thing and the demise of a number of multifunctional products.

2. **Assurance that each functionality is actually received.** The actual application of individual functional products provides potent psychological assurance that the related benefits will be provided and provided at a functional level.

3. **(Intangible) perception that superior benefits are received.** The work associated with the application of a series of products both provides "work ethic" support that superior results should be achieved and allows the users to feel they are pampering themselves.

tional products is simply based on subjective bias that cannot be reversed by the most ingenious marketing practices or advertising campaigns.* These consumers will not be swayed. It has been demonstrated that many consumers show more readiness to trust in the functionality of a series of conventional products than in that of a multifunctional product claiming to provide the same benefits. For them, "using is believing." Potential doubts about whether the second functionality of a multifunctional product really exists cannot surface when an additional product containing that functionality is actually seen, held, and applied. Similarly, potential doubts about whether the level of that additional functionality will be adequate are minimized if not vanquished through the use of conventional products.*

Cosmetologists, the professional consumers, have in many instances demonstrated their preference for conventional products. They object, primarily, to having undesired functionalities imposed on them and, at the very least, to the loss of qualitative and quantitative control of individual functionalities (Table 2) that is inherent to multifunctional products. To many cosmetologists, multifunctional products are seen to be as "professional" as a multipurpose golf club. In addition, multifunctional products have the potential to interfere with subsequent professional services, as in the case of a highly conditioning shampoo negatively impacting a permanent wave treatment. On a commercial basis, it is significant to note that cosmetologists' fees are generally based on the nature and number of services rendered. On that basis, the rendering of a series of conventional services

TABLE 2   Key Factors Negatively Impacting Selection of Multifunctional Products for Professional Use

1. **Product functionality as part of a treatment.**   As in the case of a cosmetologist shampooing hair prior to a permanent wave, unnecessary conditioning or styling ingredients could interfere with the subsequent (and in this example, the primary/major) treatment.
2. **Qualitative and quantitative control of functionality.**   The fixed ratio of the functionalities in a multifunctional product does not allow the cosmetologist to tailor the level of each treatment to the specific needs of individual clients.
3. **Practical/commercial considerations.**   Professional fees are primarily based on the number of services that are provided. Consequently, a single multifunctional service may not be seen as justifying as large a total fee as would multiple conventional services.

---

*The writer participated in a series of consumer studies in which this was determined. Temptation not withstanding, neither the groups involved nor their preferences will be identified since these studies were conducted a number of years ago and their results may no longer be applicable to the same demographic population.

would justify greater total compensation than the application of a single multi-functional product.

Counterbalancing the objections just described, truly multifunctional products offer significant convenience, efficiency, and, in some cases, a level of functionality promised but not delivered by their predecessors. Important to today's hurried lifestyle, the first two factors translate into timesaving, a factor that has been key to attracting certain groups of consumers. A prime example of this is the significant usage of two-in-one shampoos by men. Interestingly here, another advantage of this multifunctional product is that it allows some men to enjoy significant conditioning without crossing the macho barrier to the use of conditioners. (*How can this approach be employed to help men accept hair spray?*) Conversely, a moisturizing body wash could have the negative impact of depriving female consumers of the self-pampering and somewhat ceremonial step of applying body lotion.

1.3 Inherent Multifunctionality

Certain product categories routinely provide highly efficacious multifunctional benefits as the unalterable result of their chemistry. Prime examples include alcohol-containing aftershave products, where the sensation of healing is created by the same alcohol required to solubilize the fragrance; permanent oxidative hair dyes, where the hydrogen peroxide required to oxidize the dye intermediates also serves to lighten hair; and soap/syndet bars and liquid cleansing formulations, where the soap or synthetic detergent inherently provides antibacterial benefits. Indeed, consumers now expect these multiple benefits on such a casual basis that they are hard-pressed to think of these products as marvels of multifunctionality.

Ironically, a large number of permanent oxidative hair dye products pose an interesting conflict when one is considering their eligibility for classification as multifunctional products. As touched upon earlier, these products automatically lighten (or lift) the natural color of hair one to three shades while it is being colored. This is particularly apparent (and necessary) when hair is being dyed to a shade that is lighter than the original color. While the combination of this lightening action with the formula's primary function of coloring hair provides a clear example of multifunctionality, this is rarely referred to in label copy (e.g., "lightens while coloring") or exploited in advertising copy. Conversely, based upon relatively insignificant *conditioning* performance in comparison to their ability to lighten hair, such products commonly describe themselves as "conditioning color." To further complicate the issue, as already noted, such conditioning is frequently obtained through the use of a separate conditioner and/or conditioning shampoo included by the manufacturer in the product kit. Since all items in the kit can justifiably be considered to be part of the product, and the product directions instruct the use of these components, such products could conceivably be regarded as multifunctional. Again, this discussion would not subscribe to this contention, since the color mixture alone provides an inadequate level of conditioning performance. Further, the need for the use of additional conditioning components is tacitly contradictory to the contention that the primary formula is multifunctional.

2   FORMULATION CONSIDERATIONS

2.1   Preformulation Preparation

As for conventional products, the formulating chemist must consider a great number of factors in addition to formula functionality, stability, and a esthetics prior to introducing the first ingredient to the laboratory beaker. These include the following: ingredient compatibility, patent coverage/infringement, toxicology, microbiology, regulatory compliance, ingredient availability (at the required quality and cost), manufacturability, fillability, and marketing and shipping requirements. Certainly, the presence of a second functionality will further complicate a good number of these considerations, with related concerns becoming most acute for those products involving performance areas covered by over-the-counter (OTC) monographs. Complication of consumer testing, created by multifunctionality, is discussed later in this chapter.

In those cases where the combination of more than one *OTC functionality* is intended, a series of issues must be addressed, starting with the determination of whether such *crossover* is permitted by each monograph and ending with whether both monographs would permit the intended marketing claims. (For thorough discussion of such issues, please refer to the chapters in this book relating to the addition of antibacterial and sun protectant functionalities.) In those cases where an OTC functionality is to be combined with a conventional functionality, one must determine whether this will negatively impact such monograph requirements as performance-, safety-, and/or stability testing and, possibly, regulated product claims. One must also recognize that, through combination with a drug product, manufacture of what was previously a conventional cosmetic product will become governed by drug good manufacturing practices (GMPs).

Of course, the formulator must exercise a greater level of preparation prior to the formulation of a multifunctional product than is necessary for a conventional product. Given the reality that the development of a multifunctional formulation requires the establishment of an increased number of project requirements, goals, and criteria for success, it becomes that much more important for the developmental chemist to operate from the very onset of the program with a clear understanding of what is expected. Such expectations are most effectively defined, established, ratified, and communicated in a new product description document of standardized format that includes the input of the various departments involved in the project. An example of a new product description from designed for hair products was published in 1999 [2]. It is imperative that the completed new product description document include details of the desired physical attributes, aesthetic properties, functional benefits, cost parameters and, perhaps of greatest importance, criteria for success. Further, whenever possible, individual competitive (or internal) products should be cited as reference standards (or controls). Finally, to be of meaningful value, the new product description must be approved (i.e., signed) by the key decision makers in the organization.

2.2 Functional Categories

While multifunctional products may provide a virtual myriad of performance benefits, they may be thought of as falling into one of two primary functional categories (see Table 3) depending on whether the added functionality would or would not normally be expected, at any level, to be present in the parent product category. The latter category, in which the additional functionality is not expected of the parent product category, is further divided into subcategories depending on whether the added functionality is considered to be within the same functional realm as the parent product. For example, insect repellency is considered to be in a new functional realm when added to a skin moisturizer or hair spray because such functionality would not normally be associated with these products.

While each *category* comes with its own set of technological and artistic challenges, the successful amplification of a subfunctionality to a level that is adequate to be recognized as a major functionality (as in category 1, Table 3) is held in particularly high esteem by the writer. Key to this sentiment is the presumption that in achieving success, the formulating chemist was able to conquer difficulties encountered by numerous predecessors, as well as knowledge that this endeavor may have required the overcoming of a substantial functional contradiction. The

---

TABLE 3 Functional Categories of Multifunctional Products

---

1. **Significantly increased functionality of secondary performance benefit expected of that product category**
   Examples: Shampoo that conditions exceptionally well (i.e., two-in-one shampoo); body wash that imparts unusually high level of emollience (body soap with lotion).

2. **Introduction of a functionality that is not normally expected, at any level, of the parent product category**
   a. Multifunctionality within same functional realm
      Examples: dentifrice that prevents plaque; dental adhesive with antibacterial deodorant properties; moisturizing lotion that also heals
   b. Multifunctionality within new functional realm
      Examples: skin moisturizer or hair spray that repels insects; hair styling/holding products that provide UV protection

---

term *functional contradiction* refers to the common situation in which the primary functionality of the multifunctional product would normally be expected to work in opposition to the secondary functionality. For example, the primary purpose of a shampoo is to leave hair clean. In conflict with this, a conditioning shampoo, to be functional, must leave some level of residue on hair after rinsing, and this residue has the potential to be negatively regarded. A similar scenario applies to a body wash providing skin lotion functionality.

2.3 Physical Categories

In addition to classification according to functionality, multifunctional products may be placed in one of two physical categories, depending on whether they consist of a single component or two components that must be co-mixed prior to use (Table 4). Regardless of whether they are homogeneous or comprise multiple phases, products are placed in the "single-formula" category (category 1, Table 4) if they are packaged as a single component, in a single-chambered container. Homogeneity, or the lack thereof, does however impact subclassification, where distinction is drawn between products comprising a single phase or multiple phases (Table 4). With regard to the latter, it should be noted that the presence of multiple phases within a product provides an extremely effective initial signal to the consumer in support of formula multifunctionality. This remains true regardless of whether multiple phases are required to achieve multifunctionality or are present simply to impact consumer perception.

Products in the second major physical category (Table 4) consist of components that are to be maintained separately and co-mixed prior to use. Such separation of components could be required for reasons of ingredient/formula incompatibility, or could be employed to delay a desired chemical reaction until the time of product use. Similar to the case of single-component products employing multiple phases, such separation may not be required by ingredient considerations but, instead, could be employed (by multifunctional and single-function products alike) as a consumer signal. Clearly, the presence of multiple components that must be co-mixed prior to use will also reinforce consumer confidence in the presence and potency of an additional functionality. It is, however, worthwhile to note that a product is not to be considered to be multifunctional simply because its components *legitimately* require separation prior to use. Products such as baking

TABLE 4 Physical Categories of Multifunctional Products

1. **Single formula:**
    a.   Single phase (including/emulsions)
    b.   Multiple phases (e.g., layers, beads)
2. **Multiple formulas/components.**
    Require co-mixing of formulas during or after dispensing

soda–hydrogen peroxide toothpaste, hair bleach, and epoxy adhesive (not related to personal care but worthy of note) require separation of components prior to use for valid chemical reasons yet are not multifunctional.

2.4 Packaging and Dispensing Options

A number of packaging systems have been designed to sequester the component formulas of multifunctional products, yet allow them to be conveniently codispensed. They have taken a number of forms including the following: two collapsible tubes, or rigid containers, that are maintained side by side; and a single, rigid-walled container with two separate chambers (e.g., double-barreled syringe of the type commonly employed for epoxy adhesives). An overriding concern in the design of such containers is to ensure that the final unit does not become too cumbersome in size or shape to allow for ergonomically convenient dispensing.

Dispensing methods vary from the co-pouring/co-pumping of liquids from rigid-walled containers (either two containers that are maintained in tandem or a single container with two chambers), to the co-squeezing of viscous materials from collapsible tubes, to the co-extrusion of very viscous materials by plunger from a dual-chambered rigid container (e.g., system employed to dispense Chesebrough-Pond's *Mentadent* baking soda–hydrogen peroxide toothpaste [3]; the double-barreled syringe employed with epoxy adhesives). The dispensed material may vary in form, from two separate streams or ribbons dispensed in close proximity to one flow of product containing two separate streams or ribbons to one flow of product in which the streams or ribbons are co-mixed. The two latter examples require the use of a component designed to induce the material dispensed from two orifices to converge into one flow, typically a Y-shaped fitment. The final example, in which the streams or ribbons are co-mixed during dispensing, also requires the incorporation into this codispensing component of a swirl chamber or a series of baffles [4].

It is important to recognize in the design of such systems that the consumer places great conscious, or subconscious, importance on their ability to dispense the entire contents of the unit. Further, dissatisfaction in this regard cannot be assuaged by simply overfilling the product to deliver the label-stated quantity, since the consumer rarely determines the amount of product that has been dispensed. (Some marketers have taken the additional step of advising the consumer, via label copy, that the package is designed to deliver the contents stated on the label even though some product may remain in the container.) For a more comprehensive discussion of this general subject the reader is encouraged to refer to the chapter, *The Role of Packaging in Multifunctional Products.*

2.5 Codispensing Aerosols

Through the years, a variety of devices have been developed to codispense aerosolized products consisting of two liquid components that must be kept apart prior to dispensing. While the predominant commercial application of these devices has been to dispense single-function products with special features (such as self-heating shave creams, notably Gillette's Hot One), they are described in this chapter because their design principles are highly applicable to multifunctional products. It also should be noted that they were commercially employed (by Clairol) for oxidation hair dyes, which the writer considers to be multi functional (because hair is bleached during the dying process).

Garnering a great amount of industry interest during the mid-1960s and early 1970s, the earliest of such devices depended on unique valving that codispensed product from two separated sources within the same aerosol can. One source was the can itself, from which liquid was dispensed via a conventional diptube, like a conventional aerosol. The other source was a pouch (or mini-container) affixed to the valve housing, rendering its liquid contents directly available for dispensing. Liquid from each source was then codispensed at a predetermined ratio, upon actuation of the aerosol valve. One of the significant failings of these systems was their inability to maintain this predetermined dispensing ratio throughout the functional life of the unit. This had the potential to lead to product failure and to cause consumer irritation. For some formulations, it was also very difficult to prevent cross-contamination of the two liquids within the unit. Because of these issues and for a variety of other reasons, the two-source dispensing systems are no longer commercially available.

More modern attempts at codispensing aerosols have been based on the simultaneous dispensing of two separate aerosol units through a device that combines the dispensed product into a single stream. Japanese companies have commercialized several hair dye products that are dispensed (and applied) through a comb fitted to the outermost portion of the unit. A significantly improved dispensing system, whereby the contents of the two aerosol units are co-mixed via a system of baffles, has been introduced in the United States [5].

2.6   Strategic Use of Aesthetic Properties

As briefly alluded to earlier in relation to product form, a number of halo signals may be employed to encourage the purchase of multifunctional products and to reinforce consumer satisfaction with their performance. The visual presence of a second entity is likely to have the most potent impact in this regard. This second entity may be a separate phase (layer, particles, beads) within a single component product, or it may take the form of a second component. Regardless, it provides the user with seemingly concrete evidence of multifunctionality.

Further halo support may be gained through the use of fragrance, color, and viscosity as with conventional products. Among the various categories of multifunctional products, the strategic design of aesthetic properties is most difficult for homogeneous single-phase formulas (Table 4, category 1.a), since at least two

TABLE 5 Aesthetic Parameters Supporting Cleanliness for a Two-in-One Shampoo

Examples
1. **Fragrance:** citrus or evergreen bouquet
2. **Color:** maize, light blue, light green
3. **Viscosity:** lower end of acceptable range

functionalities must be considered, yet only one set of parameters may be established. Here it is necessary to decide which set of functional properties it is most judicious to support. In the case of two-in-one shampoos, where the user is frequently concerned about an undesirable conditioning residue on one hair, it may be strategically advisable to support cleanliness, as opposed to conditioning performance (Table 5). In testimony to the complexity of shaping aesthetic properties for such products, it must be noted that the parameters supporting the product's tendency to leave hair clean are, for the most part, in direct opposition to those supporting its ability to condition.

Multifunctional products that contain, or comprise, more than one entity (layer, beads, or separate components) provide the opportunity to design/employ each aesthetic attribute to reinforce the marketing position of each entity. For example, codispensed tandem tubes containing skin cleanser and moisturizer allow for the application of conventional wisdom related to the aesthetic properties of each component—with the additional requirement that they do not conflict with one another when co-mixed. Thus a white cleanser with low level of multinote/nonspecific clean fragrance might be paired with a light almond, pink, or blue moisturizer with a low level of nurturing (vanilla, almond) bouquet fragrance.

Such products also allow the use of "relative aesthetics" to support functionality. Here, for example, while both components are creams, the deployment of a relatively reduced viscosity for the cleansing component (compared with that of the moisturizing component) would tend to support its ability to clean and leave the skin free of residue. Conversely, the relatively higher viscosity of the moisturizing component would enhance the perception that it was rich in moisturizers and other beneficial ingredients. Here too, regardless of hue, a relatively lighter intensity of color would support cleansing, as opposed to moisturizing.

3 FORMULA EVALUATION

3.1 Performance Testing

The functional evaluation of formulations may be considered as a continuum, starting with instrumental laboratory evaluations and ending with consumer/market testing. The laboratory phase of this progression enjoys the greater control of environmental conditions, substrate uniformity, application parameters, test methods, and so on, and therefore provides the greatest amount of sensitivity, accuracy, reproducibility, and objectivity. Conversely, consumer testing, with less control of these parameters, provides less sensitivity, accuracy, reproducibility, and objectivity, but for many of the same reasons provides results that are more representative of real-life product usage than those gained from instrumental laboratory investigation.

Of critical importance to the evaluation of multifunctional products, and in direct contradiction to most laboratory test methods; however, consumer testing cannot evaluate individual performance properties without including the impact of other performance (as well as aesthetic) properties. In some cases this limitation is exacerbated by inherent conflicts among formula functionalities (e.g., cleansing vs moisturizing in a moisturizing body wash; cleansing vs conditioning in a two-in-one shampoo). For these reasons it is even more essential for multifunctional products than for conventional products that testing be conducted at various points of this continuum.

It is highly recommended that the evaluation of multifunctional products begin in the laboratory, where each functional characteristic may be evaluated separately on an objective basis. It is there, and only there, that the formulator can learn how well prototypes deliver each functionality (preferably in comparison with standards established in a new product description document, see Sec. 1). Then, and only if warranted by the results of these studies, testing must be conducted to determine the combined impact of the formula's multifunctional properties in the test salon and amongst consumers. Again, such testing more closely approximates the usage patterns and challenges that products encounter in real life. As is the case for conventional products, overt steps may be required to eliminate the impact of aesthetic properties on consumer-perceived performance during these studies.

As a practical note, considering the rigors necessary to conduct meaningful laboratory studies, it may be thought more convenient and expedient to bypass this phase and proceed directly to salon, clinical, or consumer evaluations. This temptation must be resisted, since without the foundation of sound laboratory-derived knowledge, this practice is likely to provide false positives or negatives based on the interference of other performance characteristics or aesthetic properties, with the result of an inferior product proceeding to market or a superior formula being discarded. It must always be remembered that if a performance-related characteristic is apparent in salon/clinical trials and/or consumer testing but is not detectable under highly controlled laboratory conditions, it probably does not exist.

3.2 Stability Testing

Of the many areas in which testing must be conducted to assure product integrity, formula stability is that most likely to be complicated by the introduction of an additional functionality. This is of particular concern because the insertion or enhancement of an additional functionality has the potential to introduce new chemical incompatibilities and to require the adjustment of the overall chemical environment (pH, ionic content, free base/acid, etc.). Further, it may become necessary to conduct functional assays for more than one parameter during the course of this testing (particularly for drug-containing formulations). Given these concerns, it is particularly important that a rigorous accelerated stability test protocol be employed [6], that samples be stringently monitored, and that negative trends and failures be promptly communicated.

At minimum, it is recommended that a formal protocol be adopted requiring the storage of samples under the following conditions with carefully documented, periodic observations as well as analytical, microbiological, and functional assays: room temperature/ambient conditions for 2 years; 45°C for 3 months (storage at 35°C for 6 months is also recommended); 5°C (refrigerator) for one year; −10°C (freezer) for 6 months. Further, a minimum of five freeze–thaw cycles should be conducted. Again, special conditions and recording procedures may be required for multifunctional products that are governed by drug requirements. (For further related information, refer to the chapters pertaining to the addition of sun protectant and antibacterial functionality to personal care products.)

4 CONCLUSION

Multifunctional formulations are likely to become increasingly sophisticated and effective as cosmetic science continues to progress. It is anticipated that increasing consumer acceptance and demand will fuel this trend as people's confidence in the (multifunctional) performance of these products grows. In short, an upward spiral in the market importance of these products is anticipated, the slope of which will be determined more by outstanding science than by outstanding marketing. Multifunctional products appear to be here to stay, and poised to grow.

In the opinion of the author, the most exciting achievements in this arena are those in which the cosmetic scientist has been able to elevate the performance of a subfunctionality to a level of such magnitude that it is perceived as creating a new product category. A prominent example, cited many times throughout this chapter, is the two-in-one shampoo. While the likelihood of attaining comparable achievements in the future may be diminished by consideration of the numbers of scientists presumed to have unsuccessfully explored these areas in the past, it is also increased by the significant strides being made on a regular basis in true cosmetic science. Prominent among these are the achievements contributing to truly efficacious skin care.

On a negative note, it is important for the marketer and scientist alike to remember (and accept) that multifunctional products may not be well received by certain individuals and demographic segments. For a variety of reasons, varying from greater belief in the functionality of single-function products to enjoying the "ceremony" of individual product application, these consumers prefer to use a series of conventional products. On the other hand, for certain demographic groups, multifunctional products may represent much more than convenience. They may indeed represent the key to the penetration of new demographic segments (e.g., the male consumer who would not use a skin moisturizer but would use a moisturizing cleanser). Extension of this phenomenon to other product areas appears to be an interesting area for exploration.

Perhaps the most effective means of convincing the new user of the multi-efficacy of a multifunctional product prior to actual trial is through the strategic deployment of product form, aesthetic signals, and packaging componentry. In addition to their traditional utility in supporting product functionality, these parameters are of great value in reinforcing consumer buy-in to product multi-functionality. Clearly, the presence of a second phase of discrete particles or beads, or an additional formula component (that must be added prior to usage) present convincing visual (and possibly tactile) reinforcement that a second functionality is present. So potent are these signals that it is likely that the consumer will gladly put up with the inconvenience of dealing with packaging systems that are somewhat more difficult to use and/or somewhat more bulky than the ideal.

It is more critical for multifunctional formulations than for conventional formulations that the full spectrum of laboratory, clinical/salon, and consumer testing be conducted. This is due to the complications that are, in most cases, introduced by the incorporation of one or more additional functionalities. Further exacerbating the situation (as discussed earlier), these additional functionalities may be contradictory to the formula's prime function. Particularly in such cases, initial testing must be conducted under carefully controlled laboratory conditions with the prime objective of separately determining whether primary performance objectives are achieved for each of the multiple functionalities. (Hopefully, such testing would have been conducted in comparison with standards that were specified in a carefully prepared new product description document.) Upon the successful outcome of this testing, prototypes must then be thoroughly evaluated by salon, clinical, and consumer test methods to determine the aggregate impact of the multiple functionalities (and aesthetic properties) under conditions of real-life usage. Here it is critical that at least one segment of this testing employ the packaging and label directions/copy intended for actual market usage.

The successful development of multifunctional products begins with the strategic deployment of the skills essential to the formulation and testing of conventional products and proceeds to higher levels of complication. In all likelihood, mastery of these complications depends on gaining an unusually thorough knowledge of formula attributes and deficiencies, as well as related consumer attitudes and usage patterns. Clearly, the development of truly multifunctional products is accompanied by negative baggage that must be fully understood and effectively dealt with to increase the likelihood of gaining consumer acceptance and, ultimately, commercial success. Given the popularity of these products, such efforts would appear to be well justified.

REFERENCES

1. Bolich Jr., R.E. et al. Shampoo composition containing non-volatile silicone and xanthan gum. US Patent 4,788,006, Nov 29, 1998; Grote, M.B. et al. Shampoo composition. US Patent 4,741,855, May 3, 1988; Oh, Y.S. et al. Shampoo composition. US Patent 4,704,272, Nov 3, 1987.
2. M Westman. Formulating conditioning products for hair and skin. In: R Schueller, P Romanowski, eds. Conditioning Agents for Hair and Skin. New York: Marcel Dekker, 1999, pp 288–292.
3. Pettengill, Multi-cavity dispensing container. US Patent 5,020,694, June 1991.
4. C. Mears et al. Applicator and dispensing device using the same. US Patent 6,168,335.
5. Arich Inc., Suite 3210, 150 Central Park South, New York, NY 10019.
6. The Fundamentals of Stability Testing, International Federation of Societies of Cosmetic Chemists, IFSCC monograph. Dorset, England: Micelle Press, 1992.

3

Multifunctional Ingredients in Hair Care Products

Damon M. Dalrymple
ABITEC Corporation, Columbus, Ohio, U.S.A.

Ann B. Toomey
Goldschmidt, Dublin, Ohio, U.S.A

Uta Kortemeier
Degussa Care Chemicals, Essen, Germany

1 INTRODUCTION

1.1 Historical Perspective or the Evolution of Multifunctional Hair Care Products

1.1.1 Shampoos

Hair care in the early part of this century strictly meant cleansing the hair, which simply translated to hair products consisting of alkaline soap. Because of such well-known drawbacks of soap as lack of lathering in hard water, deposition of calcium/magnesium soap film onto the hair shaft, and the general product form, demand for an improved product was high [1]. It was fairly common to use home treatments (e.g., vinegar, beer, lemon juice) to strip the film left by the soap on the hair [2]. In a sense, these were the first conditioning agents.

During the early part of this century, German scientist invented the first synthetic detergents. These detergents were short-chain alkylnaphthalene–sulfonate types made by reacting butyl or propyl alcohol with naphthalene followed by sulfonation [2]. The products offered a vast improvement in shampooing, providing rich lather yet easily rinsed from the hair. This resulted in more frequent shampooing. However, with the ability to fully remove sebum from the hair and thoroughly rinse the shampoo from the hair, new difficulties were noticed. The hair was now too difficult to comb as a result of tangling, and when dried, held static electricity. These difficulties led to the rapid development of the hair care market. Chemists began to carefully examine the science behind surfactants and hair care.

The original synthetic detergent was found to be extremely irritating, so researchers continued to search for a less irritating detergent. Consumers preferred rich, copious foam, and therefore the development of foam boosters began. The first were alkanolamides. Alkanolamides are prepared by reacting a fatty acid with small primary or secondary amines such as monoethanolamine (MEA) or diethanolamine (DEA). The lower fatty acids are most commonly used for shampoo formulations, cocamide MEA being the most common. The higher fatty acid chains, from DEA, demonstrate increased viscosity control. However, these diethanol amides have recently lost favor in the industry because of the possible formation of nitrosamines [3].

Formulations began to get much more complicated in an effort to capture all the desired characteristics. The use of secondary surfactants became more common. Secondary surfactants are used to improve the properties of the primary surfactants in a formulation while enhancing the performance of the final formulation. Secondary surfactants such as amphoacetates, mono- and diglyceride ethoxylates, sulfosuccinates, and betaines have long been known to reduce the irritation of primary surfactants. Betaines are by far the most common of this group. Cocoamidopropyl betaine has the ability to reduce irritation in the mucous membranes and skin, while providing a pleasant feel. Betaines also facilitate the thickening of formulations by using salt, creating very rich, luxurious foam. Another benefit of betaines is their ability to increase the biodegradation profile of a formulation. The mono- and diglyceride ethoxylates are extremely mild and improve the dermatological profile in formulations containing a primary surfactant. These molecules are excellent thickeners as well as good emulsifiers and help to solubilize many ingredients, making them a very useful tool for formulators. As a result of the many benefits these molecules bring to a formulation, they are extremely cost-effective. Quite obviously, secondary surfactants as a group are multifunctional.

1.1.2 Conditioners

Shampoos in the 1960s and 1970s contained strong anionic surfactants at neutral to slightly alkaline pH values. These shampoos were designed to strip the sebum

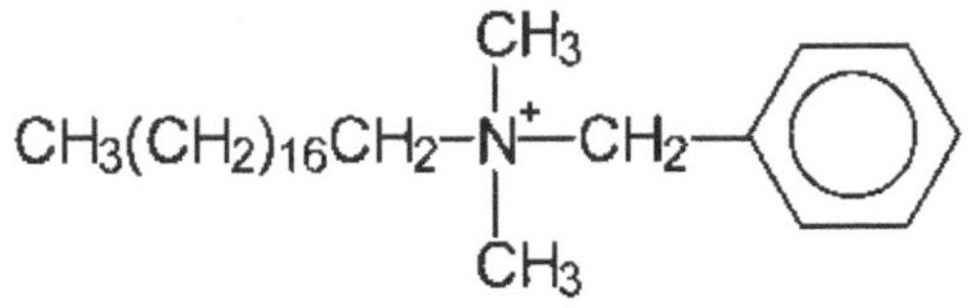

$$CH_3(CH_2)_{16}CH_2-\overset{\overset{\displaystyle CH_3}{|}}{\underset{\underset{\displaystyle CH_3}{|}}{N^+}}-CH_2-\langle\bigcirc\rangle$$

FIGURE 1 Stearalkonium chloride.

from the hair, causing the hair to tangle, as well as dulling the hair. Chemists began the search for something that would deposit onto the hair during rinsing to aid in combing and to restore luster. It was long known that quaternary ammonium compounds impart softness and static control to textiles, so it was only natural for chemists to conclude that the same would be true for hair. The first molecule to be incorporated into hair conditioners was stearalkonium chloride (Fig. 1) [4]. All quaternary ammonium compounds are similar in their chemical structure: the molecule centers around a central quaternized nitrogen atom with at least one fatty chain covalently bound. The fatty chain is what imparts the conditioning effects, more specifically, the ease of combing, the shine to the hair, and the static control. The mechanism by which this occurs is quite simple. As opposite charges attract, the positively charged cation is naturally attracted to the negatively charged hair. The quaternary ammonium compound is then substantively applied to the hair, resulting in excellent conditioning properties. Additionally, these quaternary ammonium compounds can pull further conditioning agents to the hair shaft, enhancing the deposition of silicones, oils, styling aids, and actives. Early conditioner formulations typically contained 1–2% of a quaternary ammonium compound and 5% of a long-chain fatty alcohol [1]. The fatty alcohol gave the formulation a thick creamy texture, but it also caused the hair to become limp and greasy.

The solution came in the form of Union Carbide's polyquaternium-10, a hydroxyethylcellulose derivative [1]. This molecule helped improve manageability and static control and led to a completely new raw material concept in the personal care industry. While total elimination of the fatty alcohol destabilized the formulation, reducing the amount of alcohol and replacing it with hydroxyethylcellulose improved the feel of the formulation while maintaining its texture. It improved the feel of the formulation by reducing the alcohol content, as well as imparting conditioning benefits.

Consumer demand created a new need for water-soluble cationic polymers, and many were created. These molecules had the additional benefit of increasing the deposition of water-insoluble particles on the hair during shampooing. This allowed the incorporation of zinc pyrithione in antidandruff shampoos [1]. Polymers such as polyquaternium-7, for instance, improve the deposition of antidandruff actives onto the hair during shampooing. This also opened the door for the incorporation of other functional ingredients into hair care products. Modern heat-set formulations, which improve hair manageability and hold, are now readily available from major personal care houses. Today, we even see shampoos that can temporarily color the hair.

1.1.3 Fixatives

As the frequency of shampooing increased, a wide range of hairstyles became popular, leading to the need for hair fixatives. The first hair fixatives consisted of vegetable-based, naturally isolated polymers such as quince seed and arabic gums [5]. Consumers would simply dip a comb into these products and use the comb to apply the styling aid to wet hair. The next generation of fixatives used shellac solutions in spray bottles. The difficulties with this approach are apparent: shellac is not water soluble, making its removal extremely difficult, and delivery of the product was extremely cumbersome. The next major development in fixatives came during the 1940s. The aerosol can was originally developed for dispensing insecticide [5]. A patent was issued to Goodhue and Sullivan for a low-pressure liquefied propellant. Additionally, a patent was issued to Abplanalp for a push-button valve design [5]. As a result of these patents, Kiquinet introduced the first aerosol hair spray, which allowed the use of water-soluble resins such as hydroxypropylcellulose to be sprayed onto the hair [1]. All these inventions had a profound effect on popular culture. Very high, stiff hairstyles such as the "beehive" became possible. However conditioning and styling formulations, while effective, began to lose their popularity as consumers began to notice buildup on the hair. Formulators looked for molecules that had a similar conditioning effect, but without the negative buildup. Polyquaternium-11 had long been used primarily as a fixative but had not enjoyed much popularity in the dilution–deposition era of conditioning. It was discovered that before quaternization, the precursor of polyquaternium-11 showed conditioning benefit without causing buildup [6].

1.1.4 Antidandrum Formulations

Pityrosporum ovale, a yeast, is believed to be the primary cause of seborrheic dermatitis or dandruff. It has long been known that zinc pyrithione and sulfur selenium disulfide are effective ingredients in combating dandruff. The biggest obstacle in formulating shampoos for the antidandruff market is the suspension of these active ingredients in the formulation. If not suspended properly, the active ingredient will fall out over time, resulting in an ineffective formulation [7]. The active ingredient will not properly be delivered to the scalp. The most common type of suspending agents are those that form a crystalline network in the shampoo when stationary but allow the composition to flow when shear is applied, as when shampoo is poured from a bottle [7]. An example of this type of suspending agent is ethylene glycol distereate [7]. Suspending agents of other types include cellulose gums and acrylate polymers [7]. These materials, while effective, result in an undesirable slimy feel. Another difficulty in this particular market is low foaming

[8]. Many of the antidandruff shampoos utilize coal tar as the active ingredient. These tend to be low foaming, which to the consumer means less cleaning. It is well known that foam does not equate to cleaning, but consumers prefer copious foam. Consumers also like to feel the benefit of these medicated shampoos; therefore, a cooling agent (e.g., menthyl salicylate, menthol, peppermint) is often incorporated into a formulation [8]. As a group, antidandruff shampoos exemplify multifunctionality by serving as a means to clean hair and as a delivery system for effective ingredients to relieve a medical condition.

1.2 Today's Modern Additives for Hair Care

Finally, modern polymers derived from silicones came to the forefront. They revolutionized hair care formulations. They offered many of the same conditioning properties associated with underivatized silicone, but without substantial buildup. Made from silica found in sand and quartz, silicones consist of a chain of silicon–oxygen bonds. Although silicones have become widely used in the personal care industry; there are some drawbacks: they are insoluble in water, making formulating difficult, they tend to decrease foaming, and they are greasy. Adding organofunctional groups to the silicone backbone can reduce some of these problems. These molecules are good lubricants for easy combing, both wet and dry, and they spread a smooth, even film on the hair, resulting in excellent shine and luster. Modified silicones act like surfactants in that they are surface tension suppressors, wetting agents, and emulsifiers.

2 MULTIFUNCTIONAL SURFACTANTS

The concept of multifunctionality brings to mind two separate ideas. First is the idea that a single component is able to replace many separate ingredients without sacrificing performance characteristics. Second is the concept of a single ingredient that offers varying functionality in a wide range of vastly different formulations. The latter is becoming a driving force for development, as large manufacturers are paring down their total number of inventoried raw materials. Not many single-component raw materials are able to meet this second criterion. Although there are many multifunctional ingredients, they are generally limited to specific formulations owing to their molecular functional groups, the product form of the raw material, or the functional benefit these ingredients are able to offer. To be quite simple, one would not formulate aspirin into a shampoo formulation to relieve a headache. The idea of functional availability is most important. The ingredient must function as it is intended in a large variety of formulations to meet this later definition of multifunctionality. It is not difficult to formulate low molecular weight conditioning agents into either a hair conditioner or a skin lotion. Both are emulsions differing by their function toward a substrate. What is of benefit is a single ingredient that is functional, under conditions of normal processing technology, in a wide variety of formulations. The best example of a raw material class to meet this second criterion consists of the cationic polymers such as guar hydroxypropyltrimonium chloride.

2.1 Types of Multifunctional Ingredient

Cationic polymers, originally used as film-forming fixitives, are useful in a wide variety of applications. Most are compatible with anionic, amphoteric, nonionic, and cationic compounds. Their major use remains in conditioning formulations where they improve the combing and tactile properties. They have also been shown to result in a lower irritation profile for anionic surfactants. These polymers deposit on the hair surface and impart lubricity, improving the antistatic character. Polyquaternium-7, polyquaternium-10, and guar hydroxypropyltrimonium chloride are the most common of this type. Polyquaternium-11, which is derived from poly(vinylpyrrolidone), was originally a hair fixative and has limited use in shampoo formulations. It can be argued that many of these are multifunctional additives. For this section we will focus on a select few. A detailed discussion may be found elsewhere [9].

2.1.1 Palmitamidopropyltrimonium Chloride A

The market success of multifunctional consumer hair care products has resulted in an increase in the demand for individual, multifunctional raw materials. Single ingredients that may replace multiple ingredients while at the same time adding additional functionality are gaining market share. A specific amidoamine quaternary ammonium compound, palmitamidopropyltrimonium chloride, is the best example of a single raw material that is able to replace multiple ingredients and offer additional functionality in a shampoo formulation. For example, palmitamidopropyltrimonium chloride offers conditioning, antistatic control, rheological control, and an improved dermatological profile when used in a cleansing formulation.

Amidoamine Structure and Function. This quaternary contains only two functional groups. The amido amines and their derivatives have been alkylated, alkoxylated, polymerized, and quaternized. The following example, featuring stearamidopropyl dimethylamine (Fig. 2), a very simple molecule with two functional groups, will demonstrate how a little bit of science and common sense can go a long way toward multifunctionality.

Looking at the structure one might immediately expect this molecule to function like the standard amides such as cocamide MEA. This would be a logical assumption. What is different about these two molecules? What is the same?

Cocamide MEA is used primarily in cleansing formulations. Cocamide MEA is able to affect the viscosity of formulations and to improve foam quality, stability, and flash foam. It can be perceived by consumers in the formulation by pro-

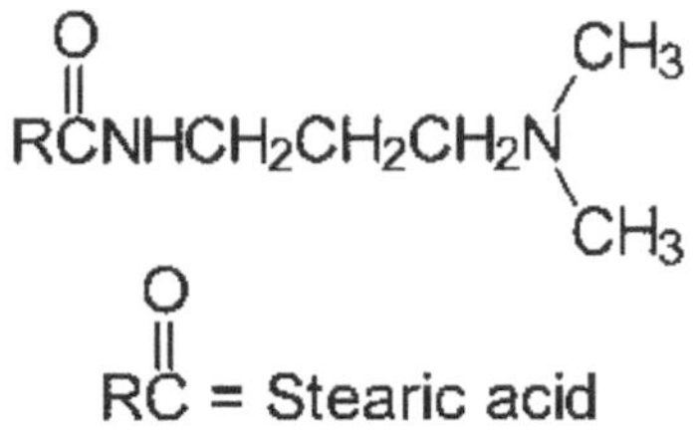

$$\overset{\displaystyle O}{\overset{\displaystyle \|}{R}} \overset{\displaystyle CH_3}{\underset{\displaystyle CH_3}{CNHCH_2CH_2CH_2N}}$$

$$\overset{\displaystyle O}{\overset{\displaystyle \|}{R}C} = \text{Stearic acid}$$

FIGURE 2 Stearamidopropyl dimethylamine.

viding a unique skin feel (refatting effect). Conversely, stearamidopropyl dimethylamine is used primarily in hair rinses and conditioners. Its primary function is conditioning (at slightly acidic pH) and emulsification. In fact, this ingredient is not easily compatible with the anionic surfactants of cleansing formulations. Stearamidopropyl dimethylamine has limited solubility in water on its own. The complex that forms with anionic surfactants is, as expected, not water soluble and must be emulsified. The base structure is very similar to cocamidopropyl betaine, the most common secondary surfactant. When stearamidopropyl dimethylamine is quaternized, either by methyl chloride, dimethyl sulfate, or diethyl sulfate, the water solubility is increased. The compatibility of this quaternary with anionic surfactants is greatly improved. Now it can be easily formulated into cleansing formulations. What is the benefit? Is there added benefit over the similar cocamide MEA offered to the consumer? The benefit is that dermatological profile, conditioning, rheological control, and antistatic behavior are all improved, as discussed in the subsequent sections. Cationics are known to vary in their ability to control static charges; however, this particular class quaternary ammonium compounds is highly effective.

Rheological Control. Further developing our cleansing formulation (shampoo), what can be done to improve the properties of this molecule? Four simple test formulations were prepared to demonstrate viscosity response versus chain length and chain length distribution of simple amido quaternaries (Table 1). All formulations were adjusted to a pH of 6.0 as is. The viscosity of these formulations was then determined (Brookfield DV II, 25°C, spindle 6 at 10 rpm) and the results given in Table 2.

Clearly, one would expect that with the actives equal, the C22 derivative of this quaternary would give the highest viscosity response. These results are, however, misleading. The chain length distribution of the quaternaries listed in Table 1 are not equivalent. These data indicate two important influences controlling viscosity: the chain length and its distribution (purity). As the chain length increases, the viscosity increases given the same purity of the distribution. The balance of the carbon count and the distribution provide the best viscosity behavior in typical cleansing formulations at C16.

TABLE 1   Test Shampoo Formulations

| | Formulations[a] | | | | | |
Ingredients	A	B	C	D	E	Purity (%)
SLES-2	12.5	12.5	12.5	12.5	12.5	
C12 DMAPA quaternary	2	—	—	—	—	98
C16 DMAPA quaternary	—	2	—	—	—	90
C18 DMAPA quaternary	—	—	2	—	—	50
C22 DMAPA quaternary	—	—	—	2	—	70
Cocamidopropyl betaine	1.8	1.8	1.8	1.8	1.8	
Sodium chloride	1	1	1	1	1	

[a]Numbers are for active ingredients.

TABLE 2   Viscosity Response vs Chain Length

Formulation	Description	Viscosity (mPa)
A	C12	38,300
B	C16	54,000
C	C18	19,000
D	C22	22,100
E	Control	300

Now we have a means of balancing the antistatic properties and the ability to build viscosity without sacrifice of either property. "Stearyl" generally refers to a broad chain length distribution centering around C18. If the carbon chain length distribution is narrowed to a pure cut, the molecule now is able to impart significant viscosity control. The foregoing example should indicate the importance of chain length distribution over carbon count for the influence of viscosity in an anionic blend. It should be noted that all the fatty acids were saturated. Substitution and unsaturation have a deleterious effect on the ability to control viscosity for this series. Ricinoleamidopropyltrimonium chloride does not build adequate viscosity in these test formulations, for instance. This idea of narrow chain length distribution also provides a significant improvement for conditioning. Additionally, for this cationic series, narrowing of the chain length improves the foam quantity and quality in formulation.

Irritation Mitigation by Palmitamidopropyltrimonium Chloride. Palmitamidopropyltrimonium chloride is an excellent emulsifier, which is substantive to hair and skin. The skin irritation index (at 30% concentration) is 0.2 (Organization for Economic Cooperation and Development Guideline 404). This is comparable to cocamidopropyl betaine, with a skin irritation index of 3.75 at 30% (Cosmetic Ingredient Review, 1995). For a low molecular weight cationic, this is highly significant. Most traditional cationics are irritants or severe irritants at this level. Additionally, palmitamidopropyltrimonium chloride has an irritation-mitigating effect on anionic surfactants. Two similar formulations were compared by means of the in vitro red blood cell (RBC) test [9]. Which measures the denaturation and hemolysis of red blood cells. This has been shown to correlate well with in vivo testing methods for irriation such as the Draize tests. The formulations are given in Table 3, which also includes the results from the RBC test. The RBC test determines a relationship between hemolysis and the percent denaturation, which is defined as the hemolysis/denaturation quotient or L/D ratio. This data can then be compared with in vivo eye data (Draize eye irritation scores). The RBC test uses a logarithmic scale (< 1 = irritant, $1–10$ = moderate irritant, $10–100$ = slightly irritant, and >100 nonirritant). It is evident that the replacement of cocamidopropyl betaine with palmitamidopropyltrimonium chloride improved the dermatological profile of this simple formulation.

Regarding substantivity in a cleansing formulation, a hand wash test was conducted with 13 panelists and the dry feel, after the hands were washed and dried, evaluated. In all cases, the subjects preferred the cleanser containing palmitamidopropyltrimonium chloride.

Conditioning of Hair.   Now we have a simple cationic ingredient that is functional in a shampoo formulation, providing the foam qualities and rheological control offered by simple alkanolamides. We also can measure an improvement in the dermatological profile of this formulation. This is all fine, but the molecule

TABLE 3   Comparison of RBC Results

	Formulations	
	1	2
SLEX-2	2.6	2.6
Disodium laureth sulfosuccinate	6.2	6.2
PEG-200 hydrogenated glyceryl palmitate (and) PEG-7 glyceryl cocoate	3.5	3.5
Sodium cocoamphoacetate	4.0	4.0
Palmitamidopropyltrimonium chloride	1.8	—
Cocamidopropyl betaine	—	1.8
RBC result (L/D)	11.0	3.2

must also function like a cationic in these surfactant systems and offer more than the traditional alkanolamides. Cationics are expected to reduce flyaway, offer conditioning, and impart excellent combing properties. The reduction of flyaway may be demonstrated by static decay measurements of individual raw materials, but logic dictates that the finished formulations be evaluated for multifunction ingredients. Figure 3 gives the static decay response times for three market-leading two-in-one shampoos with and without palmitamidopropyltrimonium chloride (Varisoft PATC) added. These data were acquired at 35% relative humidity (equilibration for 24 h) and 72°C using a Static Decay Meter (Model 401D) at 5 kV. Separate hair tresses (6 g) were stripped with sodium lauryl sulfate (SLS) (5%, aq) and soaked in the test solution (3 min) with mild agitation. The hair tresses were dried (50°C, convection oven, 1 h) and then equilibrated at constant humidity and temperature. All these formulations were improved by the addition of 1% palmitamidopropyltrimonium chloride.

Although the entire class of dimethylaminopropylamine (DMAPA) cationics provides excellent antistatic behavior, not all are compatible with anionic surfactants and offer multifunctionality. Wet comb properties vary, and many of these cationics do not give the additional benefit of rheological control and foam stability.

In hair rinse formulations, palmitamidopropyltrimonium chloride provides excellent conditioning compared with other palm-based compounds as indicated in a sensory hair tress test. Formulations F through I were prepared in water

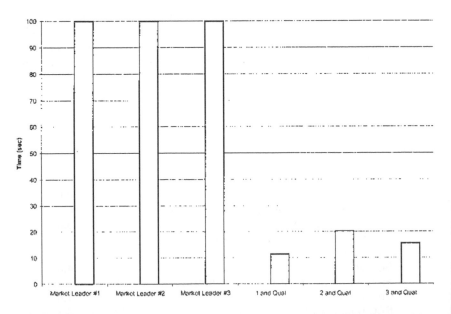

FIGURE 3 Static decay influence of palmitamidopropyltrimonium chloride.

TABLE 4 Conditioner Test Formulations

	Formulations			
INCI name	F	G	H	I
Cetyl alcohol	2	2	2	2
Quaternium-87	1	—	—	—
Dihydrogenated palmoylethyl hydroxyethylmonium methosulfate	—	1		—
PEG-3 diethylenetriamine dipalmamide	—	—	1	—
Palmitamidopropyltrimonium chloride	—	—	—	1
Ceteareth-20	1	1	1	1

TABLE 5 Results of Sensory Test for Wet Properties

	Formulations			
	F	G	H	I
Feel on hair	1.5	2	3	4.5
Rinsability	2.5	2	4	4
Detangle	5	5	2	5
Wet comb	3.5	4	3.5	4.5

(actives are given) and the pH adjusted to 4 (Table 4). These formulations were then evaluated in a sensory hair tress test (Table 5). Typically, the hair tress test must be conducted in blind, using several panelists. Under these conditions, statistical difference may be determined and a salon test followed to ascertain the laboratory results. For these simple test formulations, no salon test was conducted; however, the differences for the wet properties are apparent. These palm derivatives were evaluated on a scale of 1 to 6 (6 was best).

It has been shown that palmitamidopropyltrimonium chloride is an antistatic agent. Figure 4 gives the static decay response times for several traditional quaternary ammonium compounds with similar structures. The chemical structures of these molecules are given in Fig. 5. From these data, one would deduce that the static decay response time is a result of the amide functional group. To demonstrate this, several analogues of palmitamidopropyltrimonium chloride were synthesized and assayed for static decay. All these cationics had static decay response times comparable to that of palmitamidopropyltrimonium chloride.

One would then expect that the comparable stearamidopropyl dimethylamine at low pH would give a similar result. This, however, is not the case. The

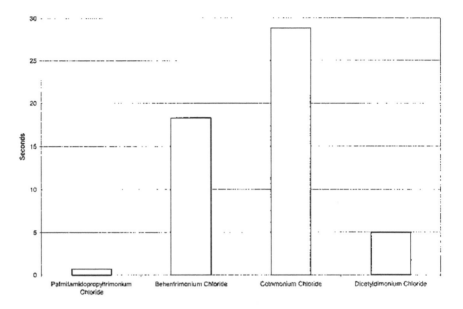

FIGURE 4 Static decay of traditional cationics.

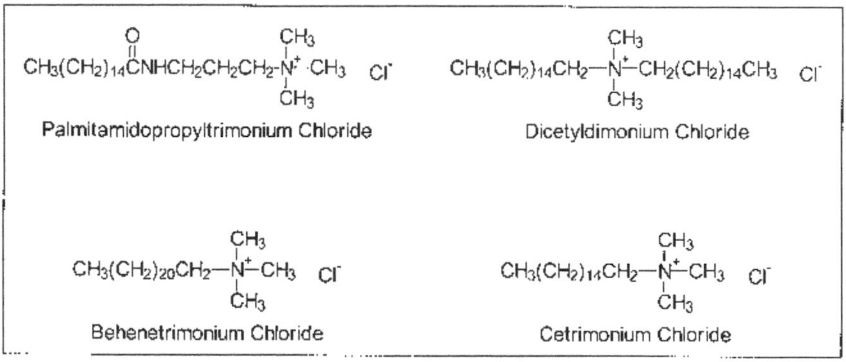

FIGURE 5 Chemical structures of traditional cationics.

inductive effects of the additional methyl group of the quaternaries gives a much stronger cationic character to the nitrogen than does simple protonation. This is also evidenced in the combination with anionic surfactants.

Stearamidopropyl Dimethylamine at low pH is not able to form a functional complex with SLES, whereas the amido quaternaries are. Regarding the solubilizing properties of amido quaternaries, the chain length distribution has a profound effect. Palmitamidopropyltrimonium chloride is able to form a microemulsion of oil in water, whereas the comparable ricinoleamidopropyltrimonium chloride and other similar amidoquaternaries listed in the Cosmetic Toiletry, and Fragrance Association (CTFA) Dictionary are not. This gives additional formulation possibilities.

The rheology of palmitamidopropyltrimonium chloride is also uncharacteristic. The viscosity of a simple blend (actives: 12% SLES, 2% palmitamidopropyltrimonium chloride, 1.8% NaCl) at pH 6.0 increased from 4780 cP at 20°C to 7800 cP at 30°C. Additionally, when dilute aqueous solutions of palmitamidopropyltrimonium chloride are heated in the presence of anionics, the water may gel. This gel is thixotropic, however, and the rheology is returned to normal with simple stirring. Therefore, this molecule is capable of providing some unique formulation rheology.

2.1 Functional Ultraviolet Absorbers in Hair Care

Many consumer shampoos with traditional UV absorbers are currently marketed around the world. These shampoos claim UV protection for hair. It is generally recognized that because of their water insolubility, these traditional UV absorbers are not readily deposited onto the hair during shampooing. Because shampoo formulations are different from sun-screen formulations, these molecules are really not suitable for shampoo applications. To improve the substantivity of UV absorbers, quaternary ammonium functionality has been combined with UV filters in a single molecule. Two excellent examples follow.

Dimethylpabamidopropyl Laurdimonium Tosylate B. The damage caused to hair by ultraviolet radiation is well known. Tryptophan degradation, cystine residue reduction (weakening the strength of the hair), and changes of the cuticle all are recognizable as damage induced by UV light [10–13]. Although commercially available sunscreens are able to protect against UV-A and UV-B light, they are not functionally suitable for hair care. In cleansing formulations, typical sunscreens are not substantive toward hair. It is not difficult to realize that they were not designed for rinse-off applications. In conditioning formulations, these ingredients are water insoluble and also lack substantivity.

The degree of sun damage to hair tresses was indirectly measured through a staining method with a Hunter Lab Colorimeter. Comparison of treated and untreated hair tresses using thiol-indicating Merbromin stain demonstrated significant protection of the hair shaft with dimethylpabamidopropyl laurdimonium tosylate (as Escarol HP-610 from ISP) [19]. Approximately a 50% improvement was measured [14]. In an additional study measuring the photoprotection of tryptophan a 25% increase in tryptophan stability was measured by means of fluorescence spectroscopy [14,15]. To further demonstrate the protection offered by dimethylpabamidopropyl laurdimonium tosylate, a combing test was performed with a Diastron Miniature Tensile Tester. Three standard sunscreens (octyl methoxycinnamate, DEA methoxycinnamate and benzophenone-3) were compared with dimethylpabamidopropyl laurdimonium tosylate. The test products were applied to damaged hair as solutions. After rinsing, the hair tresses were irradiated for 72 h. The tresses were then shampooed to eliminate any surface treatment effects. Comparative measurements were then taken. The results are given in Fig. 6. The surface damage was reduced for the sample treated with dimethylpabamidopropyl laurdimonium tosylate.

Cinnamidopropyltrimethylammonium Chloride C. Cinnamidopropyltrimonium chloride was introduced to the hair care market in 1998 (Fig. 7). Cinnami-

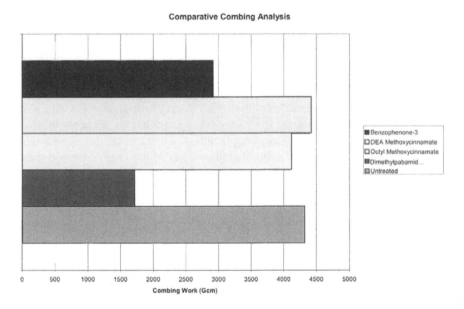

FIGURE 6 Coming force measurements.

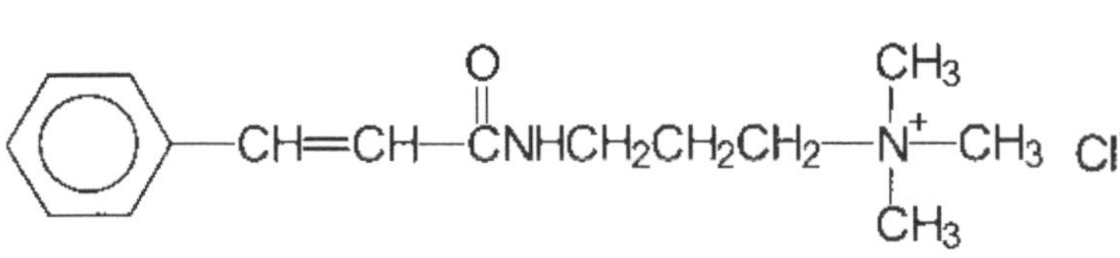

FIGURE 7 Cinnamidopropyltrimonium chloride.

dopropyltrimonium chloride has a molar extinction coefficient of 21,605 cm^2/mol at 280 nm[1] [16]. It is a liquid at room temperature and easy to process. Because sunscreens vary in their water solubility they often are diluted by perspiration. Consistent reapplication of sunscreen is often needed. Another obstacle to overcome is the need to provide substantivity without overloading the hair shaft. Preparation of sunscreen formulations employing hydrophobic carriers may result in a product having unfavorable properties such as a greasy feel. This is a particular problem for formulation for hair care and protection. Cinnamidopropyltrimonium chloride is an amidoquaternary that is water soluble yet at the same time highly substantive toward hair. To demonstrate the deposition of the cationic onto hair, a standard rubine dye test was conducted using bleached hair. A 2% w/w active aqueous solution was compared to a blank of deionized (DI) water. This standard technique gave a positive response to the hair tresses with cinnamidopropyltrimonium chloride [16].

It has been shown that cinnamidopropyltrimonium chloride is able to protect blonde hair from damage by UV radiation. Two simple cleansing base formulations were compared. Both contained 10% SLS. One contained 2% octyl methoxycinnamate (an approved sunscreen in the United States) and the other, 2% cinnamidopropyltrimonium chloride. Bleached blonde hair tresses were treated with both formulations and then subjected to light in the UV-B range. A third untreated hair tress was also subjected to UV-B light. A fourth hair tress, used as a positive control, was not subjected to UV-B radiation. The results clearly showed a degradation of color for the untreated hair tress and the hair tress treated with octyl methoxycinnamate solution. The hair tress treated with cinnamidopropyltrimonium chloride and the hair tress not subjected to UV-B light were virtually identical [17].

2.1.3 PEG-200 Hydrogenated Glyceryl Palmate (and) PEG-7 Glyceryl Cocoate D

The multifunctional properties of certain polyethylene glycols (PEG-200 and PEG-7) include rheology control, solubilization, emulsification, foam density improvement, irritation mitigation, and tactile feel improvement [18]. This blend is capable of replacing alkanolamides in shampoo formulations without a sacrifice of performance properties. In addition, the dermatological profile is improved [18]. This blend of glyceride ethoxylates is prepared by transesterification of the whole oils with glycerine followed by ethoxylation (200 and 7 mol on palm and coco, respectively). The end products are then blended in a ratio of about 70:30 to provide balanced multifunctionality in a single product. Figure 8 gives the salt curves for 2% thickener [as PEG-200 hydrogenated glyceryl palmate (and) PEG-7 glyceryl cocoate or cocamide DEA], and 12% SLES-2 in water.

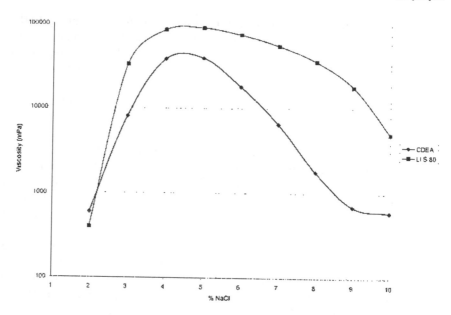

FIGURE 8   Salt response curve for CDEA and Li S-80.

2.1.4   Disodium PEG-5 Laurylcitrate Sulfosuccinate E

An ingredient that offers excellent cleansing and foaming in shampoo formulations while improving the dermatological profile of the formulation is disodium PEG-5 laurylcitrate sulfosuccinate E, which also has the potential to replace alkanolamides in shampoos based on ammonium lauryl/laureth sulfate.

As commercially available, disodium PEG-5 laurylcitrate sulfosuccinate is an extremely mild surfactant that scores zero on the Draize test (Fig. 9). It offers mild cleansing and a good foam volume. It is an excellent emulsifier and offers a pleasant skin feel. Figures 10 and 11 give comparative results of an in vitro irritation test (the RBC test, described earlier) for two simple ternary surfactant blends. These figures compare the combination of an alkylpolyglucoside (APG), ethoxylated mono- and diglycerides, and sodium laureth sulfate compared with the same blend replacing APG with disodium PEG-5 laurylcitrate sulfosuccinate. The dermatological profile is improved when one is formulating with disodium PEG-5 laurylcitrate sulfosuccinate instead of APG. Specifically, the combination 80:10:10 in Figs. 10 and 11, respectively, clearly show the improvement in dermatological properties—moving the classification from "Irritating" to "Moderately Irritating" by simply replacing the alkylpolyglucoside.

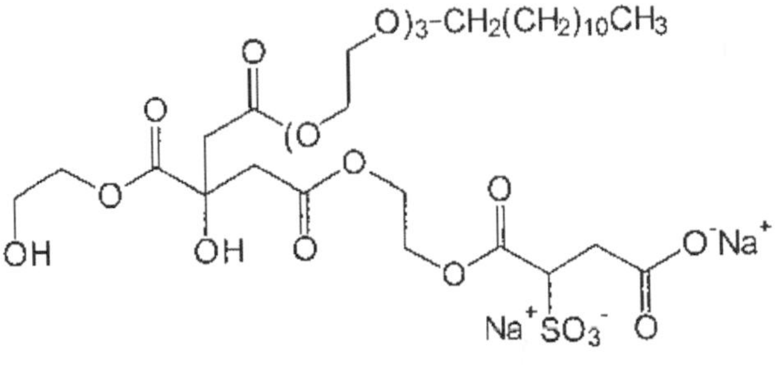

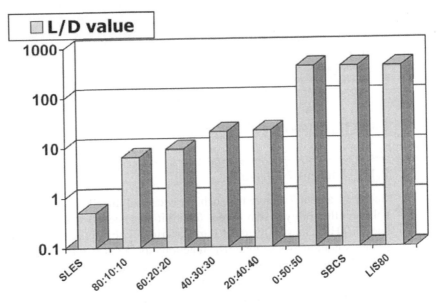

FIGURE 9 Disodium PEG-5 laurylcitrate sulfosuccinate.

FIGURE 10 Ternary blends with disodium PEG-5 laurylcitrate sulfosuccinate.

It is well known in the art that sulfosuccinates as a chemical class pose drawbacks in formulation regarding rheological control. This particular sulfosuccinate; however, when formulated with ammonium-based salts, such as ammonium laureth sulfate and ammonium lauryl sulfate, builds excellent viscosity. The viscosity response with salt (ammonium chloride or sodium chloride) results in viscosities up to 35,000 cP at a pH of 6.

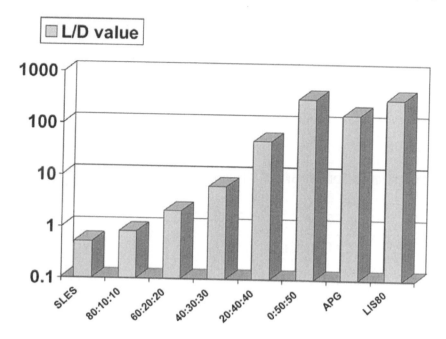

FIGURE 11   Ternary blends with alkylpolyglucoside.

2.1.5   Laureth-7 Citrate F

Because Laureth-7 Citrate has such a low critical micelle concentration (cmc), it enhances the ability to remove oils (conditioning agents) and sebum from hair (at specific pH). It may be formulated into a stripping shampoo or directly into a two-in-one conditioning shampoo. The functionality of this surfactant is pH dependent and offers much versatility. Because this surfactant is diprotic, the emulsification properties are easily adjusted with pH. It is possible that at low pH, the deposition of conditioning agents and actives onto the hair shaft is improved.

Laureth-7 citrate is a commercially available liquid at 99% solids (Fig. 12). in vitro RBC data, indicate that it is an extremely mild secondary surfactant with excellent emulsifying properties. It functions as a dispersing and suspending agent, is low foaming (Ross–Miles pH 7, 60 mm), and offers the added benefit of oil removal from skin and hair. A simple formulation of laureth-7 citrate at 2% is able to emulsify 8% mineral oil. The same level of laureth-7 citrate is able to disperse walnut shell powder at 5% for a peeling cream. It is able to form stable emulsions with insoluble additives. It has a dispersion efficiency of 3.5 g for 80% insoluble matter in water. Laureth-7 citrate is a solubilizer for natural oils such as lavender oil, pine oil, and rosemary oil, and is able to form clear systems.

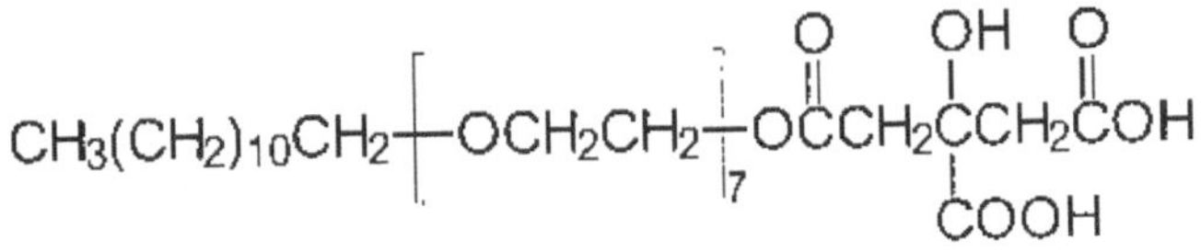

$$CH_3(CH_2)_{10}CH_2 \left[OCH_2CH_2 \right]_7 O\overset{\overset{\displaystyle O}{\|}}{C}CH_2\overset{\overset{\displaystyle OH}{|}}{\underset{\underset{\displaystyle COOH}{|}}{C}}CH_2\overset{\overset{\displaystyle O}{\|}}{C}OH$$

FIGURE 12 Laureth-7 citrate.

The sequestering properties were investigated by Diez et al [19], who found a chelating value expressed as molar efficiency of 23–27% [19]. Clearly, there is some sequestering ability for this surfactant; however the efficiency is low.

To study the oil-removing (cleansing) properties of laureth-7 citrate, a cleansing test was performed in which fabric served as a model. The fabric was impregnated with silicone oil (dimethicone) and washed with a 5% surfactant solution. The fabric was dried, and gravimetric analysis of the oil removal was assayed. The results are given in Fig. 13 for the three surfactants tested (sodium laureth-3 sulfate, disodium PEG-5 laurylcitrate sulfosuccinate, laureth-7 citrate, and water as a blank). Laureth-7 citrate offers deep cleansing and is recommended in shampoos for greasy hair. Its extreme mildness and its ability to remove dimethicone efficiently make possible an additional benefit in two-in-one formulations, namely, the prevention of buildup.

Furthermore, when the static decay method described earlier was used, Laureth-7 citrate gave a surprising result of 6.76 seconds. This was highly unexpected and may be explained by the same hydrogen bonding mechanism described next for is the diacetyltartaric acid ester of glycerol monostearate (INCI name: DATEM).

2.1.8 Laureth-3 (and) DATEM F

Suitable in shampoo formulations for enhanced body and manageability, DATEM offers improved combing properties while enhancing the deposition of conditioning additives or actives.

Food additives are a natural choice for cosmetic ingredients owing to their excellent toxicological profiles. DATEM, food additive that has proven itself functional in cosmetic formulations, provide improvement of combability, detangling, and feel for both wet and dry hair. It is now confirmed through Fourier transform infrared (FTIR) studies that DATEM associates with proteins through hydrogen bonding of the polar amino acid residues and the carbonyl groups of DATEM as shown in Fig. 14, a schematic representation of the association of DATEM and the protein structure of hair. The normal absorption frequency is shifted by 2.5 cm^{-1} with a weakening of the carbonyl peak clearly evident as well.

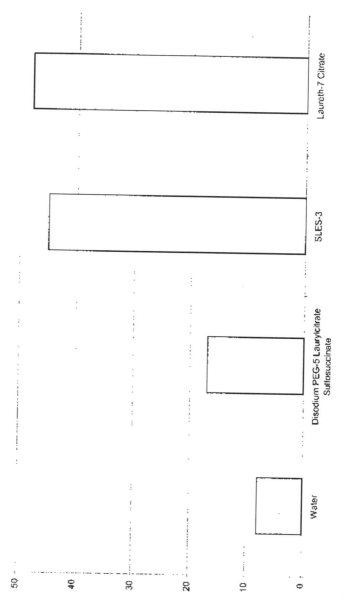

FIGURE 13   Percent oil removal by surfactants.

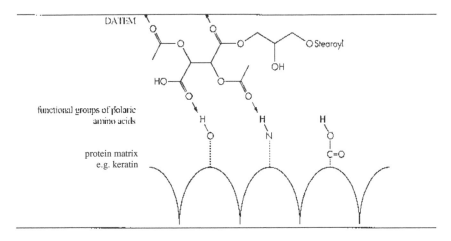

FIGURE 14 Schematic representation of DATEM association with hair.

Others have shown DATEM to provide excellent conditioning properties in shampoo formulations [20,21]. Further studies conducted by Kortemeier and Leidreiter demonstrated improvement in the dry properties for a simple shampoo formulation [10% SLES (actives) and 0.4% DATEM] over the same formulation with substitution of 0.2% polyquaternium-10G or just SLES [22]. For the wet comb, the formulation with polyquaternium-10 was superior to all others.

In a half-head test done by a hairdresser with 20 subjects, the wet feel and the elasticity of a shampoo containing only 0.4% DATEM was preferred in comparison to control. Also the dry combability was judged to be slightly better.

In a second hair swatch test, the formulations of Table 6 were evaluated. For all properties but shine, the differences were dramatic. The formulation with 0.5% DATEM (formulation 2) provided an improvement of up to 33% in most cases over the formulation containing 1.0% (formulation 3) or the formulation with no DATEM. Formulation 2 provided better feel and combability and, in particular, improved the detangling properties of wet hair (Fig. 15).

The three formulations also were compared with respect to curl retention, and the data surprisingly showed a benefit to formulation 2, containing 0.5% DATEM. This formulation improved the curl retention by approximately 10% in comparison to the blank (Fig. 16). These identical formulations were then tested separately by subjects who had either fine hair or thick hair (Fig. 17). The results were quite different and highly significant. For subjects with fine hair, formulation 2 was judged to be better in an in-use consumer test. The results of the test group with thick hair were entirely different, however. Formulation 3 was highly preferred in this case. With this study it is recommended that DATEM be used for fine

TABLE 6   Shampoo Formulations

	Formulations (%)		
	1	2	3
SLES	32.1	—	—
CAPB	8.0	—	—
Laureth-3	1.5	—	—
DATEM	0	0.5	1.0
Perfume	0.1	—	—
TEGO® Pearl N100	1.0	—	—
Water	To make 100.0	—	—
NaCl	0.4	0.6	0.82

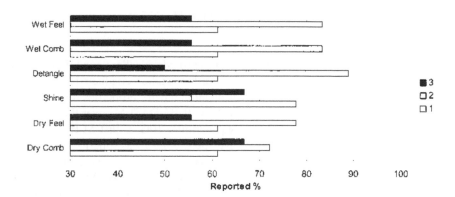

FIGURE 15   Results of half-head test.

to normal hair. For these hair types, improved soft setting and volumizing effects were measured. The dry feel was improved and the curl retention was improved significantly.

3   ORGANOMODIFIED SILICONES

Organomodified silicones, in shampoo formulations, offer improved foaming characteristics and combing properties, as well as improved deposition of care ingredients onto the hair. These ingredients are excellent as emulsifiers and solubilizers, which offer additional substantivity toward hair.

From the initial incorporation of dimethicone into cleansing formulations and conditioners for hair, consumer demand for silicone functionality has grown.

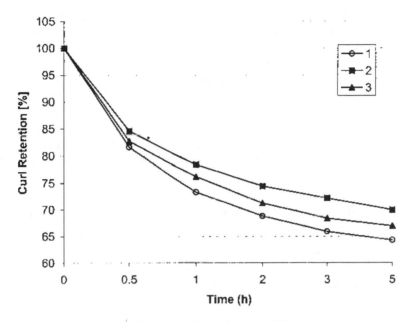

FIGURE 16 Curl retention at 70% relative humidity.

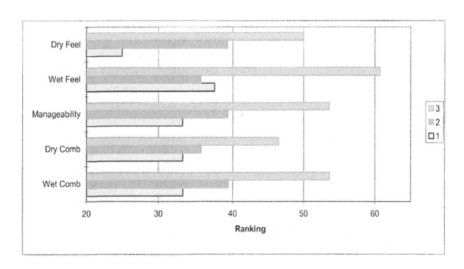

FIGURE 17 Results of hair swatch test for thick hair.

This created additional demand for silicone derivatives that are multifunctional. The basic backbone remains the same (Si—O—Si); however, the options for derivatization range from simple pendent alkyl chains to complex α, ω-polyalkoxylated structures with additional functionality such as quaternized nitrogen or amines. Modified silicones provide increased performance through enhanced substantivity, increased emulsion stability, better shine, increased wetting time, and improved rheological control and film-forming deposition properties on hair. These properties are directly related to the type of functional group substituted and the mole percent of this substitution on the backbone. The main silicone derivatives to be discussed are the alkyl siloxanes, dimethicone copolyols and quaternary silicones.

3.1   Alkyl-Modified Silicones

Modified silicones are easier to handle and offer greater functionality and versatility. The particular class of alkyl-modified silicones (cetyl dimethicone) offer improved formulation stability in addition to film-forming properties and increased spreading rates. As is often the case, alkyl-modified siloxanes were not developed for the cosmetic industry, but borrowed from an industrial application [23]. Like many raw materials, they were adapted to suit the cosmetic industry. They are prepared by substitution of an alkyl group on the linear polydimethylsiloxane (PDMS) backbone. The physical form of this class of raw materials ranges from oils low in viscosity to high melting solids. Naturally, this is dependent upon the alkyl chain length, its distribution, branching, and degree of substitution, in addition to the properties of the polymer backbone. These materials do not give the typical greasy properties of organic waxes. They impart thickening for most emulsion types and give body and cushion to the end formulation. The polymeric backbone is responsible for the loss of greasy tact and substitutes the typical "silicone" feel [24]. The alkyl moeity is responsible for formulation stability, flexibility, and compatibility with organic additives.

The synthesis of organosilicone water-in-oil emulsifiers is based upon the linkage of polymethylsiloxane chains with alkyl side chains and polyglycol groups. The polymethylsiloxane chain possess both hydrophilic and lipophilic characteristics. The polyglycol groups provide the necessary hydrophilic characteristics, and the side chains provide lipophilicity. The performance properties may be easily adjusted by varying the side chain, the siloxane backbone, and the ethylene oxide/propylene oxide content. The high functionality of these materials is likely due to the strong absorption at the phase boundaries. The requirements of multifunctional hydrophobic emulsifiers are best provided by polymeric materials. These requirements are easily met by the polyalkyl polyether polysiloxane copolymers. They are active at a level of 1–3% and form very thin interfacial films. They are highly flexible toward interfacial stress.

One class of lipophilic emollients of particular interest is the polyalkyl polysiloxane copolymers. It is known that polyalkyl-modified polysiloxanes are compatible with emollients, waxes, and other silicone polymers. They are excellent additives for improving the slip properties of emulsions. Simple combination of a variety of examples from this class with typical emollients such as isopropyl myristate, octyl stearate, and caprylic/capric triglycerides were compared for their spreading. The addition of 0.1% w/w of cetyl dimethicone (as ABIL Wax 9840) reduced the surface tensions of simple emollient esters by 20%, for instance. Furthermore, the uniform deposition of traditional actives and quaternaries onto hair is improved by these alkyl-modified siloxanes [24].

3.2 Cationic Polydimethyl Siloxane

Incorporation of cationic or amphoteric groups into the copolyol leads to increased substantivity toward polar substrates. This provides the deposition of a durable film onto the surface of the hair shaft. Polydimethylsiloxanes modified with cationic groups combine a high gliding ability with marked antistatic properties. Polyether side chains may also be included in addition to the ionic groups to improve the solubility and compatibility in formulation.

Silicone quaternary compounds provide excellent conditioning with the added benefit of mildness. This is a feature not generally shared with their traditional counterparts (quaternary ammonium compounds). Since the silicone quaternaries are relatively expensive, they are not used widely as replacements, but rather as additives (0.2–0.4%), to improve the tactile properties.

Quaternium-80 is a diamidoquaternary polydimethyl siloxane somewhat intermediate between traditional quaternary ammonium compounds such as palmitamidopropyltrimonium chloride and silicones (Fig. 18). This molecule combines the best of both worlds. The excellent static control property of amido quaternaries is retained, as well as the film-forming properties of silicones. In addition, quaternium-80G is compatible with anionic surfactants, making it highly suitable for two-in-one shampoos. The charge density of quaternium-80 is much lower than that of traditional cationics, however. This can be easily overcome through combination. Several similar hair rinse formulations were prepared and

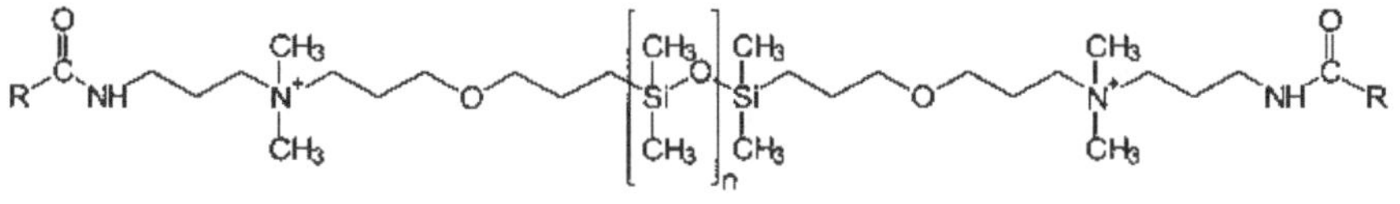

FIGURE 18 Quaternium-80.

assayed for the performance properties. These included sensory evaluations, half-head tests, wet and dry combing force measurements, volume force measurements, and gloss determination. The active components of conditioning agents were kept at 2.0%.

First, a hair swatch test was used to compare sensory conditioning properties such as wet comb, dry comb, dry feel, and flyaway behavior using the test formulations of Table 8. Both, virgin Caucasian (European) bundled hair (2 g weight, 18 cm length) and virgin Asian (Chinese) bundled hair (3 g weight, 18 cm length) were purchased (Kerling, Germany). The hair tresses were subjected to predamage by means of permanents and bleaches using trade standard products (Wella). Tap water (37°C, 8°dH = 80 mg CaO/L H_2O) was used to wet the hair. One gram of test formulation was then applied to each hair tress, and carefully worked into the tress. Following an action period of 1 minute, the hair was rinsed with tap water (37°C, 8°dH) for 1 minute After the excess water had been pressed out with a towel, the wet hair was assessed directly by means of a precisely defined system of criteria. This system of assessment criteria gives assessment marks for each characteristic property. Here, "5" designates an excellent assessment, "1" means that there is deficiency. Following an assessment of wet comb, the hair tresses were dried overnight at 25°C and 50% relative humidity in a hanging position. The same system of assessment criteria was again used to assess the dry comb and dry feel. The results of the test with Caucasian hair showed that cetrimonium chloride, stearamidopropyl dimethylamine, and the combination of stearyldimethylamine and quaternium-80 gave comparable conditioning results [25]. Independently, the formulation with quaternium-80 alone does not appear to perform as well as the cationics for the property of dry comb [25]. On Asian hair, the test formulas performed similarly except that a small advantage was noted for the combination of stearamidopropyl dimethylamine and quaternium-80 [25].

In addition to the sensory test performed on hair tresses, the shadow contour method was used to indirectly measure the static charge on the hair tresses [25]. This test was performed at constant temperature and humidity. Each hair tress was hung in front of a concentric measuring scale. A single point light, at a defined distance, was used to project the shadow of the hair tress. The hair was charged by defined combing and the shadow contour measured for each hair tress. The results for both Caucasian and Asian hair are given in Fig. 19.

All test formulations gave similar responses with the exception of quaternium-80 on Asian hair. This may be explained by the difference in charge density of the silicone derivative in comparison to the traditional molecules. The performance of quaternium-80 on Caucasian hair may be explained by a film-forming lubrication effect rather than by antistatic behavior due to charge [25]. Because Asian hair is more structured and thick, the effect of the silicone is not as dramatic.

Furthermore a half-head test with a trained hairdresser was carried out on the foregoing formulations. For that cetrimonium chloride (CTAC) was compared

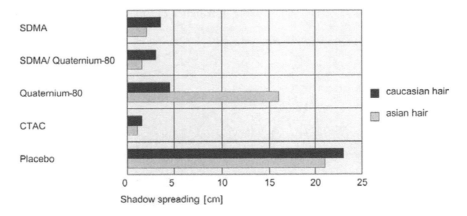

SDMA

SDMA/ Quaternium-80

Quaternium-80

■ caucasian hair

☐ asian hair

CTAC

Placebo

0   5   10   15   20   25

Shadow spreading [cm]

FIGURE 19   Flyaway by shadow contour method.

with stearamidopropyl dimethylamine (SDMA) quaternium-80, and the combination according the properties shown in Fig. 19. Between CTAC and SDMA no statistical difference for all tested parameters was found. Quaternium-80 gave a significantly better wet combability and an arguably better gloss. The results of the combination compared to CTAC are given in a radial graph (Fig. 20). Specifically, the wet comb property was enhanced for the combination (quaternium-80 and stearamidopropyl dimethylamine), rather than for the single ingredients [25].

The body/volume force of quaternium-80 toward hair was assayed in accordance with a standard method [26]. All formulations in Table 7 were tested with this method. The results indicated that quaternium-80 was equivalent to a standard cationic for reduction of body (Fig. 21). Quaternium-80 and CTAC reduced the body force measurements the most significantly. This is further evidence for the deposition properties of quaternium-80.

3.3 Polyether Polysiloxanes

Typically, polyether polysiloxane copolymers have pendent structures (Fig. 22). In these copolymers, the performance that is expected from the silicone moiety is often masked. The silicone backbone is free to rotate, while at the same time the repeating polyether is free to wrap around the silicone backbone. This may explain the lack in performance of these materials in comparison to the α,ω-derived copolymers (Fig. 17). A new dimethicone copolyol was prepared by using the silicone backbone of quaternium-80 and derivatizing α and ω with a 40:60 ratio of ethylene oxide to propylene oxide (Fig. 23) [27]. This structure was selected based upon the surface tension measurement of several analogues in aqueous sodium

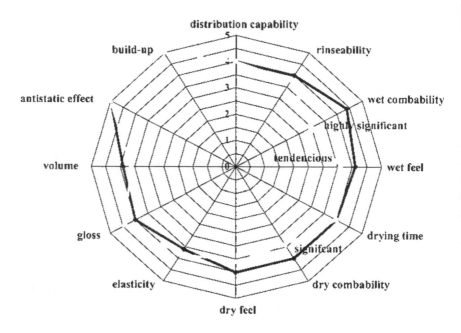

(5 = excellent; 1 = very deficient)   CTAC ➡ SDMA/Quaternium-80

FIGURE 20 Comparative results from salon test.

TABLE 7 Active Ingredients in Test Formulations[a]

	Active ingredients (%)				
	CTACl	SDMA	Quaternium-80	SDMA/quaternium-80	Placebo
Ceteareth-25			0.5		
Cetyl alcohol			2.0		
CTAC	2.0	—	—	—	—
SDMA	—	2.0	—	1.0	—
Quaternium-80	—	—	2.0	1.0	—
Water	To make 100.0%				
	pH 4.0 ± 0.2				

[a]CTACl, cetrimethylammonium chloride; SDMA, stearamidopropyl dimethylamine.

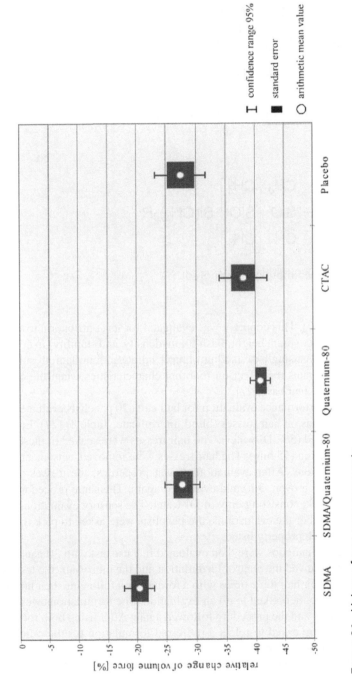

FIGURE 21 Volume force measurements.

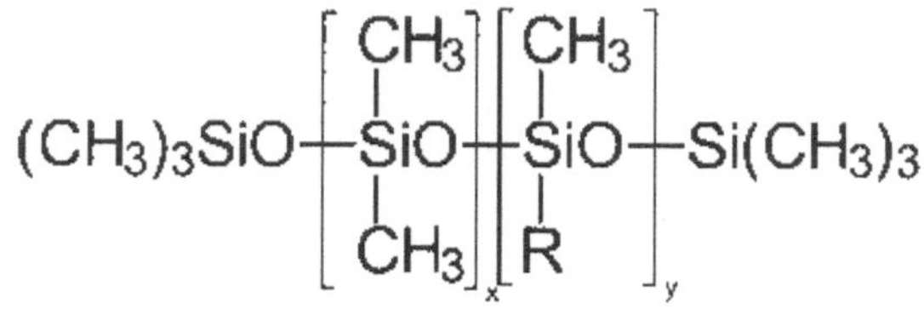

$$(CH_3)_3SiO \left[\begin{array}{c} CH_3 \\ | \\ SiO \\ | \\ CH_3 \end{array} \right]_x \left[\begin{array}{c} CH_3 \\ | \\ SiO \\ | \\ R \end{array} \right]_y Si(CH_3)_3$$

FIGURE 22   Pendent type of modified siloxane.

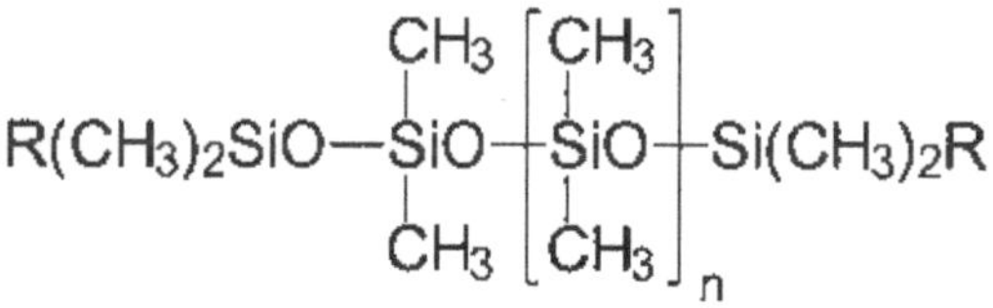

$$R(CH_3)_2SiO - \begin{array}{c} CH_3 \\ | \\ SiO \\ | \\ CH_3 \end{array} \left[\begin{array}{c} CH_3 \\ | \\ SiO \\ | \\ CH_3 \end{array} \right]_n Si(CH_3)_2R$$

FIGURE 23   New dimethicone copolyol.

lauryl sulfate [27]. This copolyol was evaluated for its contribution toward foaming characteristics (foam height, flash foam, density, and stability) in combination with a simple cleansing base (sodium lauryl sulfate/sodium laureth sulfate). Figure 24 demonstrates the effect on foaming characteristics when the copolyol is added to a surfactant base [27].

For the performance evaluation for hair care, 20 panelists evaluated two separate formulations on hair tresses (blind, in triplicate, Table 8) [27]. Each formulation was diluted (5%, DI water). The hair tresses were soaked in these solutions with mild agitation (15 min). The hair tresses were removed, rinsed, and hung for the wet evaluations. After evaluation of wet properties, the tresses were dried (40°C, convection oven, 3 h) and evaluated again. The same procedure was followed for a blank, consisting only of DI water. The sensory evaluations are given in Table 9 [27]. For the evaluations, the panelists were asked to pick the best formulation for each property listed.

The two shampoos were then evaluated in a use test with 20 panelists. Half the panelists received the control formulation and the other half, the test. All panelists washed their hair three times with a formulation following their normal daily routine and were then asked to do an evaluation. The formulations were reversed to eliminate bias and the procedure followed again. After using both formulations, the panelists were asked to select a preferred formulation for the criteria of wet comb, wet feel, dry comb, and so on (Fig. 25). These results indicate an advantage to the formulation containing the new dimethicone copolyol (ABIL® B 8832) for

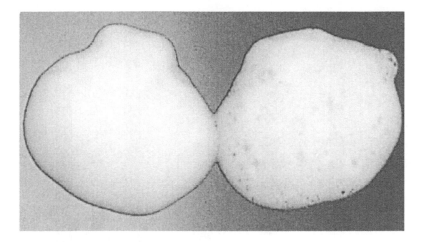

FIGURE 24 Foam generated through a foam valve.

TABLE 8 Test Formulations

Ingredients	Control (wt %)	Test (wt %)
Water	47.9	47.4
Tetrasodium ethylenediamine-tetraamine	0.1	0.1
Ammonium laureth sulfate	25.0	25.0
Ammonium lauryl sulfate	15.0	15.0
Cocamidopropyl betaine (and) lauryl glucoside	10.0	10.0
PEG-18 glyceryl oleate/cocoate	2.0	2.0
Experimental copolyol	—	0.5
Ammonium chloride	q.s.	q.s.
Total	100.0	100.0

all properties except clean rinse, where neither formulation offered a clear advantage [27].

POLYQUATERNIUM-10 AND POLYQUATERNIUM-46

Polyquaternium-10 is recognized as the leading multifunctional ingredient for hair care today. It is widely used in a variety of formulation ranging from cleansers to hair fixatives. Polyquaternium-10 is easily formulated, offering improved deposi-

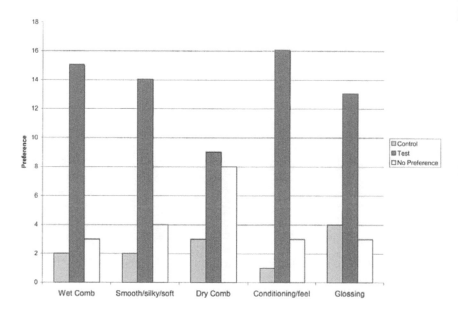

FIGURE 25   Preference rankings for half-head test.

tion of care ingredients toward hair. It was the first cationic polymer offered in a shampoo formulation.

Its deposition on hair is dependent upon the type of surfactant present. Non-ionic and amphoteric surfactants facilitate greater deposition, whereas primary anionic surfactants give a weaker substantivity. It is used in permanent waves, conditioning shampoos, body washes, and shower gels, and hair rinses and conditioners. One must be careful in formulating with polyquaternium-10, as it is known to build up onto the hair shaft. The properties it imparts to hair are improvement in wet and dry comb and reduction in flyaway.

Polyquaternium-46 offers improved curl retention without sacrifice of combing properties. Like other cationic polymers, this polymer is suitable in a wide range of formulations for hair care while retaining its intended functionality—improved manageability.

Polyquaternium-46 is a newer multifunctional ingredient for hairstyling formulations. This fixative is suitable for modern water-based formulations that are free of volatile organic compounds. It has a charge density much lower than other polyquaterniums (0.5 mequiv/g) [28]. In spite of this, the conditioning properties are quite good. Like other cationic polymers it is compatible in shampoo formulations. Polyquaternium-46 provides a greater reduction in combing force than polyquaternium-16 and polyquaternium-11. The curl retention effects were

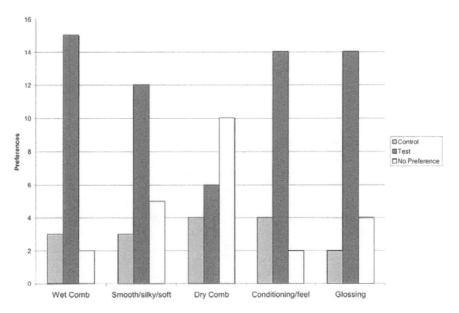

FIGURE 26 Preference rankings for sensory evaluations.

assayed at 75% relative humidity for polyquaternium-11, 16, and 46 and also PVP/MA copolymer. Polyquaternium-46 was superior to all of these and additionally had measurable benefit even at 90% relative humidity [28].

CONCLUSION

From the examples given in this chapter, it should be evident that a variety of chemically distinct, multifunctional raw materials are available to the formulator. Time and space prevented the inclusion of many other multifunctional materials; but the examples used demonstrate the possibilities available. Although most consider polymers to be multifunctional, this convention does not preclude nonpolymeric materials from this classification. If demand for multifunctional consumer products continues, the number of new multifunctional raw materials will naturally increase. Compatibility and synergism with active ingredients combined with the functional availability of individual raw materials is the key to success. Demand for highly functional individual ingredients that offer additional benefits is driving raw material producers toward multifunctional ingredients. The future is a practical one, where personal care products can do more with less. Regarding the environment and resources, having single ingredients, which can replace multiple raw materials, is a benefit for everyone.

REFERENCES

1. Urbano CC. 50 Years of hair-care development. Cosmet Toiletries 110(12):85–104 (1995).
2. Encyclopedia Britannica. Soap and detergents, 1999.
3. Reiger M. Surfactants in shampoos. Cosmet Toiletries 103(3):59–72 (1988).
4. US patent 4,610,784.
5. Walls E, Krummel HK. Low VOC hairsprays: Formulation challenges for a changing industry. Cosmet Toiletries 108(3):111–117 (1993).
6. Lochhead, RY. History of polymers in hair care (1940–present). Cosmet Toiletries 103(12):23–54 (1988).
7. Woodrow T. International Patent PCT/US96/00295, July 25, 1996 Procter & Gamble Co.
8. Fang H. International Patent PCT/US98/02731, Feb 6, 1998, Procter & Gamble Co.
9. Domsch A, Irrgang B, Moeller C. Mild surfactants—Facts and illusions. SOFW J June 1996, p 122.
10. Speakman JB, MacMahan PR. The action of light on wool and related fibers, N Z J Sci Technol, 20:2488 (1939).
11. Milligan B, Tucker DJ. Studies on wool yellowing. III: Sunlight yellowing. Text Res J 33:773 (1963).
12. Holt LA, Milligan B. The involvement of tryptophan in the photoyellowing of wool. J Text Inst 67:269 (1976).
13. Tolgyesi E. Weathering of hair. Cosmet Toiletries 98:29–33 (1983).
14. http://www.ispcorp.com/products/hairskin/haircare/p0er13.html. June, 2000.
15. US Patent 5,427,773.
16. US Patent 5,601,811, 1997.
17. http://www.croda.com.
18. Egan R. Ethoxylated mono and diglycerides as nonionic surface active agents and anti-irritants. Annual Meeting of the Society of Cosmetic Chemists, May 1982.
19. Diez, Park, Fique, Alkyl ether citrate surfactants. CESIO, 1996.
20. Leidreiter HI, Jorbrandt C, Jenni K. Comparative evaluation of modern conditioning agents by tests on hair tresses. SOFW J 120:852–860 (1994).
21. Leidreiter HL Mueller F. Verwendung der Diacetylweinsauerester von Fettsauereglycereiden als Haarkonditioniermittel. DE PS 44 08 668, 1974.
22. Leidreiter HI, Kortemeier U Glycerol esters of tartaric acid give conditioners specific properties. In press.
23. US Patent 3,416,353.
24. Floyd DT, Howe AM Alkyl-modified siloxanes: Key ingredients for formula optimization. Formulation Forum '99, Orlando, FL, March 3–5, 1999.
25. Kortemeier U, Leidreiter HI. Conditioning properties of stearamidopropyl dimethylamine: Sensory assessment and technical measurements. PCIA-2000.
26. Robbins CR, Crawford RJ. Method to evaluate hair body. J Soc Cosmet Chem 35:852–860 (1984).
27. Floyd DT, Leidreiter HI. A new novel silicone copolymer for personal care product. Unpublished paper.
28. Hoessel P. A new multifunctional polymer. Cosmet Toiletries 111 (August 1996).

4

Multifunctional Shampoo: The Two-in-One

Michael Wong*

Clairol, Inc., Stamford, Connecticut, U.S.A.

1 INTRODUCTION

The two-in-one shampoo, also known as a conditioning shampoo, or one-step shampoo, is the most common type of multifunctional shampoo. It performs the dual function of cleaning and conditioning hair in a single step. Over the years, the two-in-one shampoo has grown in popularity and consumer acceptance, and has become a significant component of the shampoo category.

The appeal of this important shampoo segment is the convenience the product has to offer. The two-in-one replaces the typical combination of shampoo and postshampoo conditioning treatments. It eliminates the extra steps and the tussles of having to reach for another bottle of conditioner in the middle of shampooing and rinsing your hair. It has indeed addressed an important consumer need.

The considerable success of the two-in-one in the marketplace is the ability of the product to deliver the expected performance benefits, in spite of the technical challenges of having to combine the two hair care regimens that are potentially incompatible or even mutually exclusive. This chapter explores the two distinct processes involved in hair cleaning and hair conditioning, and also reviews the advances of this two-in-one technology over the years.

---

*Retired

2   HAIR CLEANING VERSUS HAIR CONDITIONING

A two-in-one shampoo has the dual functions of cleaning and conditioning hair at the same time. Hair cleaning and conditioning are two processes that operate on entirely different principles. They are expected to provide different benefits to the hair, and they require ingredients with significantly different properties.

2.1   Hair Cleaning Aspects

Functioning as a shampoo, a two-in-one should provide sufficient detergent actions to remove all the "unwanted" hair soil, which consists of hair lipids [1–7], dust particles [8], skin debris [9] from the hair shaft, and all other residues from previous hair cosmetics, such as hair spray. Shampoo removal of hair soil is a complex process [10–20], requiring the use of ingredients that are highly surface active. The cleaning agents should be able to wet the hair surface thoroughly. They should have the required properties to help emulsify and to solubilize the hair soil to facilitate its separation from the hair.

Shampooing also requires the production of desirable lathering characteristics that users tend to equate with hair cleaning. Effective shampoo ingredients must be able to develop a dense and copious lather. They must be highly water soluble and rinse off easily, without leaving any residues on the hair.

The materials that meet these requirements are anionic surfactants. Anionic surfactants are substances that carry a negative ion and contain both an oleophobic moiety and a hydrophilic moiety in the same molecule. They are soluble in water and are highly surface active. In aqueous solutions, at a concentration above the so-called critical micelle concentration (cmc), they tend to form micellar structures that are believed to be essential to the solubilization and emulsification processes that pull the soil particles from the hair surface. For these reasons, anionic surfactants are the cleaning ingredients of choice in shampoo formulations.

Amphoteric surfactants are also used in shampoos to some extent. These are compounds that have two different ionic sites on the same molecule. One of the ionic sites, which is cationic, can be amino nitrogen or a quaternary compound. The anionic site is either a sulfate, a carboxylate, or a sulfonate [21]. The surfactant as a whole can be cationic, anionic, or zwitterionic, depending on the pH of the medium. The amphoteric surfactants generally do not clean as well or lather as effectively as anionic surfactants. But they are found to be milder [22,24], and interestingly, when mixed with anionic surfactants, they are tend to act synergistically to lower the level of irritations of the latter [23].

Hair cleaning action does have some consequences on hair aesthetics. Thoroughly cleaned hair has both wanted and unwanted attributes. Shampoo removes the hair soil and leaves the hair shiny and lustrous. It restores hair body. But thoroughly clean hair also feels raspy and harsh. Additionally, it is difficult to comb through. It is prone to static buildup that tends to generate excessive flyaway, making the hair hard to manage.

2.2 Hair Conditioning Aspects

Hair conditioning is, in a sense, hair cleaning in reverse. In contrast to shampooing, which involves the removal of materials from the hair surface, conditioning is the action of putting back onto the hair an appropriate amount of suitable ingredients. While shampoo relies on the actions of anionic materials, hair conditioning requires the use of materials that are different in every aspect in terms of ionic characters, surface properties, and solubility characteristics.

One requirement of an effective hair conditioning agent is a proper degree of substantivity to the hair. The conditioning agent in a two-in-one shampoo must be able to survive the detergent actions of the cleaning agents as well as the subsequent rinsing actions. Another requirement is that the conditioning agent be able to impart to the hair the desirable tactile properties. Hair conditioning is expected to make the hair feel soft and smooth, to make the hair easy to comb, and to prevent static buildup. The amount of conditioning residues must not be excessive, which can create the phenomenon of "overconditioning," causing limp, dull-looking hair that is difficult to style.

Effective hair conditioning agents are in general cationic. They are more oleophobic, and are much less soluble in water. The ones that are commonly used are quaternary ammonium compounds, cationic polymers, and silicon oil. The substantivity of cationic materials is due to strong ionic interactions between the positive charges and the negatively charged hair surface. The substantivity of silicone oil, on the other hand, is a result of hydrophobic interactions. Being oleophobic, these conditioning agents also tend to suppress foam production and to have adverse effects on the lathering characteristics of anionic surfactants, complicating the task of formulating the the two-in-one shampoos.

Quaternary ammonium compounds are materials that contain at least one nitrogen atom with four alkyl or aryl groups attached to it. These compounds are always cationic regardless of the pH of the medium, and for this reason are in general not compatible with anionic surfactants.

Cationic polymers are materials made by attaching quaternized fatty alkyl groups to synthetic polymers or to modified natural polymers. Some quaternized polymers are extremely substantive to hair surface because of the high charge density. They are compatible or incompatible with anionic surfactants depending on the structures of the polymers and more importantly on the proportions at which the two are combined.

Silicone oils are also good, effective hair conditioning agents. They are highly hydrophobic and sparingly soluble in water. They are typically incompatible with anionic surfactants and need to be emulsified in a special way.

3 FORMULATING TWO-IN-ONE SHAMPOOS

The essence of the two-in-one shampoo technology is to incorporate the appropriate conditioning ingredients into a shampoo base to achieve both cleansing and conditioning of hair in one step from a single product. For the conditioning agent to work properly in a shampoo formula, it must be not only substantive to the hair but strong enough to survive the accompanying detergent actions and the subsequent water rinse. Equally important, it should have minimal interference with cleansing actions or lathering characteristics. These were challenges that confronted earlier chemists [25–28]. But thanks to the stream of new or improved ingredients, a clear understanding of the properties and interactions of these materials, formulation strategies have evolved over the years and in fact have become more routine. The advances of this technology are discussed next.

3.1   The Cationic/Amphoteric Combinations

A typical approach to formulating one-step conditioning shampoo in the late 1960s and early 1970s was to incorporate a hair conditioning agent into a shampoo base consisting primarily of amphoteric surfactants. A number of such agents were reported, including protein hydrolysate [29] and mineral oil [30]. The materials most frequently used, however, were monomeric quaternary ammonium compounds [33,34] or quaternized polymers [31,32]. These are cationic materials that contain quaternary nitrogen to give them unusual substantivity to the hair surface [35,36]. The quaternary ammonium compounds, especially those with a long alkyl chain (14–22 carbons), have been known to be able to impart some unique properties [37–39] to the hair and have been widely used in hair rinse conditioners. They have been claimed to make the hair feel soft and smooth, easy to comb, and less prone to static buildup. Taking advantage of these ingredients, formulators had some success in formulating one-step shampoo by utilizing quaternary compounds in combinations with amphoteric surfactants. A typical example of such a formulations is shown in Table 1. The choice of amphoteric surfactants was primarily dictated by concerns that cationic and anionic materials would not be compatible, and that either cleansing or conditioning would be severely compromised.

TABLE 1   Shampoo Formulation with Amphoteric/Cationic Combination

Ingredients	Amount (wt %)
Cocoamphodiacetate	20.00
Coamidopropyl hydroxysultaine	12.00
Glycerol stearate	1.00
Lauramide DEA	3.00
Hydrolyzed protein	2.00
Polyquaternium-27	2.40
Deionized water	As needed to make 100

Source: Ref. 40.

This novel concept of a one-step shampoo was well received. It generated a lot of consumer interest and had considerable impact in the marketplace, with Milk Plus Six (from Revlon) as the prime example. The success was short-lived, however, because of some inherent shortcomings. It became increasingly apparent that the hair cleansing action was not sufficient, and there was slow buildup of residues on the hair. On repeated usage, these shampoos would "over condition" the hair, leaving it limp, weighed down, and lacking in body. Again, formulators began refocusing their efforts to develop a one-step shampoo using anionic surfactants as the primary cleaning agents. The amphoteric/cationic combinations alone are rarely used these days. Practically all the two-in-one shampoo formulations contain some anionic surfactants.

3.2 The Dilution–Deposit Technology

An important milestone for the two-in-one shampoo takes advantage of hair conditioning attributes of some cationic polymers and some unusual mixture properties of cationic polymers and anionic surfactant. Cationic polymer and anionic surfactant paired in a single system would normally be incompatible, producing an insoluble complex that would precipitate. It was found, however, that at some ratio of surfactant to cationic polymer, when the surfactant is in excess, the precipitate could be redissolved to form a clear solution. What is important is the concentration of the anionic surfactant. When the anionic concentration is above its cmc, the complex is solubilized to form a stable emulsion. But if the anionic concentration is brought below its cmc, the complex will become insoluble and precipitate. This phenomenon was first observed by some researchers who quickly recognized its implications as a useful "trigger mechanism" to deliver conditioning from shampoo formulated with anionic surfactant. The idea was that when the cationic and anionic surfactant are formulated appropriately, the complex should stay dissolved in the shampoo but precipitate onto the hair surface when diluted with water upon rinsing. This discovery spurred a flurry of research activities [30,41–46] and patent disclosures [47–51]. Indeed, this technology has evolved into a major strategy to formulate two-in-one shampoos. Some typical formulations are shown in Tables 2 and 3.

3.3 The Silicone Advantages

Another important advance in the two-in-one technology was the utility of silicone polymers as hair conditioning agents in a shampoo. The appeal of silicone was the rather unique surface properties that cationic surfactants and quaternized polymers did not have. Silicones were found to be able to impart certain dry conditioning attributes to the hair that the polymer–surfactant complex cannot deliver as effectively. The molecular structures and flexibility [54] of some silicone polymers are believed to promote unusual lubricity of the hair and to make the hair feel

TABLE 2 Shampoo Formulation Using Cationic Polymer with
Anionic Surfactants

Ingredients	Amount (wt %)
TEA lauryl sulfate (40% active)	38.00
Lauramide DEA	3.00
Hydroxyethylcellulose	1.00
Polyquaternium-11	2.00
Hydrolyzed protein	2.00
Perfume/preservatives	As needed
Deionized water	As needed to make 100

Source: Ref. 52.

TABLE 3 Shampoo Formulation Using Cationic Polymer with
Anionic Surfactants

Ingredients	Amount (wt %)
Cocoamphodiacetate/disodium cocamido sulfosuccinate	18.50
TEA lauryl sulfate (40% active)	18.50
Propylene glycol	2.00
Lauramide DEA	4.00
Polyquaternium-10	0.70
Citric acid	0.50
Preservative/fragrance	As needed
Distilled water	As needed to make 100

Source: Ref. 53.

soft and smooth. The low surface tension and high refractive index of these polymers allow them to improve hair shine and luster [55]. In fact, numerous patent disclosures dating back to the 1960s claim the uses of silicon polymers as effective conditioning agents for shampoo [56–63]. Silicone polymers, however, are highly hydrophobic, and have limited solubility in water or other common organic solvents. The challenge of having silicones in shampoo formulations was not only to keep the various ingredients properly suspended but to ensure that they remained stable over the shelf life of the product. The answers to this challenge were revealed by the patents issued to Procter & Gamble [61,62]. In these patents, the company has claimed a unique formulation technology and manufacturing process for a shampoo composition containing nonvolatile silicones, anionic surfactants, and other ingredients to achieve a stable and emulsion; moreover, the silicone is said to have minimal effect on shampoo lather and cleansing. It works by depositing on hair via dilution upon rinsing. This technology became the basis of Pert Plus and other two-in-one shampoos across P&G's product line. Subsequently, Vidal Sassoon, Pantene, Ivory, and Head and Shoulders all have taken this major technological advance and used it to improve product performance across the board on a large front. In response to this development, other shampoo manufacturers have also mounted major efforts to match or surpass this patented technology, resulting in a flurry of product launches [64], as well as research and patent activities [65–71]. Some typical examples of two-in-one shampoos formulated with silicons are shown in Tables 4 and 5.

3.4 Using Both Cationic Polymers and Silicone

As the two-in-one technology has further evolved, formulators are beginning to use a blend of cationic polymers and silicones as dual conditioner in two-in-one shampoos. One advantage of this approach is that the two conditioning agents are complementary. While the polymer–surfactant complex gives the hair excellent wet conditioning effects, silicones provide superior dry benefits, imparting unusual silkiness and softness to the hair. Another advantage is that this approach offers a considerable degree of formulation flexibility. The combination would avoid using excessive high concentration of either the cationic polymers or silicones. Too much polymer–surfactant complex would have the potential to cause a

TABLE 4 Shampoo Formulation Using Silicone Polymer with Anionic Surfactants

Ingredients	Amount (wt %)
Ammonium lauryl sulfate (40% active)	16.00
Xanthan gum	0.75
Cocamide MEA	2.00
Dimethicone	1.00
Cetearyl alcohol	1.00
Silicone gum	1.00
Fragrance	1.00
Sodium chloride	0.10
Preservatives	0.03
Caustic soda (50% active)	0.01
Ethylene glycol	0.75
Dye solution	0.65
Water (double reverse osmosis)	As needed to make 100

Source: Ref. 62.

TABLE 5 Shampoo Formulation Using Silicone Polymer with Anionic Surfactants

Ingredients	Amount (wt %)
Ammonium lauryl sulfate (40% active)	16.00
Ammonium lauryl-3-sulfate	4.00
Ammonium xylenesulfonate	2.20
Cetearyl alcohol	1.00
Glycol distearate	0.75
Cocamide MEA	1.00
Xanthan gum	0.75
Dimethicone	1.00
Silicone gum	1.00
Tricetyl ammonium chloride	1.00
Fragrance/color	As needed
Water	As needed to make 100

Source: Ref. 72.

slow buildup of residues. Too much silicone in a shampoo would severely affect the lathering characteristics. Thus, this approach has become a useful tool to formulate a two-in-one product that is able to clean hair adequately and is also able to deliver the best of hair conditioning characteristics. The key is to recognize the appropriate combinations of cationic polymer, silicone, anionic surfactants, and amphoteric surfactants. In fact, a recent survey of 10 different major commercial brands shows that the majority of two-in-one shampoos are now formulated almost exclusively using both cationic polymers and silicones as conditioning agents. The essential ingredients of these brands are summarized in Table 6.

4   SHAMPOO COMPONENTS

The key ingredients required to formulate two-in-one shampoos, discussed in the subsections that follow, are hair cleaning agents, hair conditioning agents, foam boosters, and preservatives.

4.1   Hair Cleaning Agents

In spite of the large number of detergent surfactants are now available, only a handful are the bread-and-butter cleaning agents used in the majority of two-in-one shampoos, or even in shampoo products in general. Formulators tend to pre-

TABLE 6 Functional Ingredients in Commercial Two-in-One Shampoos in Year 2000

Ingredients	Commercial brands of two-in-one shampoos									
	A	B	C	D	E	F	G	H	I	J
Anionic surfactants										
Sodium (or ammonium) lauryl sulfate	×		×	×	×		×	×	×	
Sodium (or ammonium) laureth sulfate			×	×	×	×	×	×	×	×
Sodium cetearyl sulfate	×									
Sodium trideceth sulfate		×								
Sodium carboxylate		×				×				
Sodium lauroyl sarcosinate				×						
TEA-dodecylbenzenesulfonate									×	×
Disodium ricinoleamidosulfosuccinate					×					
Amphoteric surfactants										
Coco betaine	×									
Cocamidopropylhydroxysultaine		×								
Disodium lauro(or coco)-amphodiacetate		×			×	×				
Cocamidopropyl betaine									×	×
Silicone polymers										
Dimethicone	×		×	×		×		×	×	×
Amodimethicone							×			
Quaternized polymers										
Polyquaternium-10		×	×	×	×	×	×			
Polyquaternium-15						×		×		
Guar hydroxypropyltrimonium chloride	×								×	×
Hydroxypropyltrimonium hydrolyzed protein	×									
Nonionic surfactants as foam booster or emulsifer										
PEG-150 distearate (or glycol distearate)		×	×	×		×	×	×		
Cetyl alcohol (or lauryl alcohol)			×	×			×	×		
Hydrogenated polydecene			×							
Cocamide MIPA (or cocamide MEA)			×				×	×		
Glyceryl palmate (or cocoate)	×				×	×				

fer the ingredients that have a long history of safe use, perhaps out of concerns about efficacy, costs, or regulatory issues. The typical cleaning agents commonly found in the two-in-one shampoos are alkyl sulfates, alkyl ether sulfates, alkyl sulfonates, alkyl benzenesulfonates, sulfosuccinates, sarcosinates, betaine, amphodiacetate, and hydroxysultaine, as described next.

4.1.1 Alkyl Sulfates and Alkyl Ether Sulfates

Two anionic surfactants are used exclusively in the majority of two-in-one shampoos today, frequently serving together as a blend. These are alkyl sulfates and alkyl ether sulfates. The alkyl sulfate is represented by the following structure:

$$R\text{--}O\text{--}SO_3M$$

where R is an alkyl of 12 carbons or 14 carbons, and M is a cation such as sodium, ammonium, or triethanolamine (TEA).

The alkyl sulfates often found in the two-in-one shampoos are sodium lauryl sulfate, ammonium lauryl sulfate, or TEA lauryl sulfate, each with its limitations. Sodium lauryl sulfate, for example, does not have good aqueous solubility at low temperature, while ammonium sulfate needs to be formulated at low pH, and TEA lauryl sulfate has a tendency to hydrolyzed at acidic pH.

The alkyl ether sulfates are milder surfactants than the alkyl sulfates, and are less irritating to the eyes. But their lathering and viscosity characteristics are inferior. This is why they are often used in blends with alkyl sulfates to take advantages of the benefits of each surfactant type. The alkyl ether sulfates has the following chemical structure,

$$R\text{--}(OCH_2CH_2)_n\text{--}O\text{-}SO_3M$$

where R is an alkyl chain with 12–14 carbons, and n is the degree of ethoxylation, usually between 1 and 5.

4.1.2 Alkyl Sulfonates and Alkyl Benzenesulfonates

The sulfonates as a class have some useful shampoo and detergent characteristics. They are anionic surfactants that have excellent "flash" foam, superior cleaning power, and stability over a wide range of pH values [73]. But they also have negative properties that keep them from being used more widely. The alkylbenzene sulfonates, for example, tend to be more irritating to the eyes. The alkyl sulfonates are believed to have difficulties with viscosity control and consistency among different suppliers, or even among different batches from the same supplier [74]. The chemical structures representing the sulfonates are

$$RCH=CHCH_2SO_3M \quad \text{(Alkene sulfonate)}$$

and

$$RCH(OH)CH_2CH_2SO_3M \quad \text{(Hydroxy alkane sulfonate)}$$

where R is an alkyl chain with 12–14 carbons, and M is a cation such as sodium.

4.1.3 Alkyl Sulfosuccinate and *N*-Acyl Sarcosinates

Alkyl sulfosuccinate and *N*-acyl sarcosinates are also anionic surfactants that are occasionally found in two-in-one shampoos but not used as primary cleaning agents. They foam poorly and do not have the required detergent power, but they very mild and believed to have some hair conditioning effects. Also, they are more compatible with the cationic conditioning agents. Examples of these surfactants are disodium monococamido methylisopropylaniline (MIPA) sulfosuccinate, disodium-monolaurylsulfosuccinate, sodium lauryl sarcosinate, and cocoyl sarcosinate.

4.1.3 Betaine, Amphodiacetate, and Hydroxysultaine

Amphoteric surfactants also used some formulations of two-in-one shampoos include betaine, amphodiacetate, and hydroxysultaine. They are typically formulated in combination with one other anionic surfactant, because amphoteric surfactants by themselves do not have superior cleaning power or lathering characteristics. However, they are exceptionally mild for surfactants, and have very low level of eye irritations. They are also believed to work synergistically with anionic surfactants to lower the overall eye irritancy [22,23]. Examples of amphoteric surfactants often used in two-in-one are cocamidopropyl betaine, disodium lauroamphodiacetate, and cocamidopropyl hydroxysultaine.

4.2 Hair Conditioning Agents

Quaternized polymers and silicone polymers are the two categories of conditioning agents most commonly found in the two-in-one shampoos. Very often they are used in together to take advantage of their combined hair conditioning benefits.

4.2.1 Quaternized Polymers

The quaternized polymers suitable for formulating two-in-one shampoos are polyquaternium-10 (polymer JR), polyquaternium-11 (Guafquat), polyquaternium-7 (Merquat 550), guar hydroxypropyltrimethylammonium chloride, and polyquaternium-15. Polyquaternium-10 is a polymeric quaternium ammonium salt of hydroxethylcellulose. Polyquaternium-11 is quaternary ammonium polymer derived from diethyl sulfate and a copolymer of vinyl pyrrolidone and dimethyl aminoethylmethacrylate. Polyquaternium-7 is a polyquaternium salt from the reactions of acryamide and dimethyl diallyl ammonium chloride. Guar hydroxypropyltrimethylammonium chloride is polysaccharide quaternized with hydroxypropyltrimonium chloride. The chemical structures of these polymers are as follows.

Polyquaternium-10:

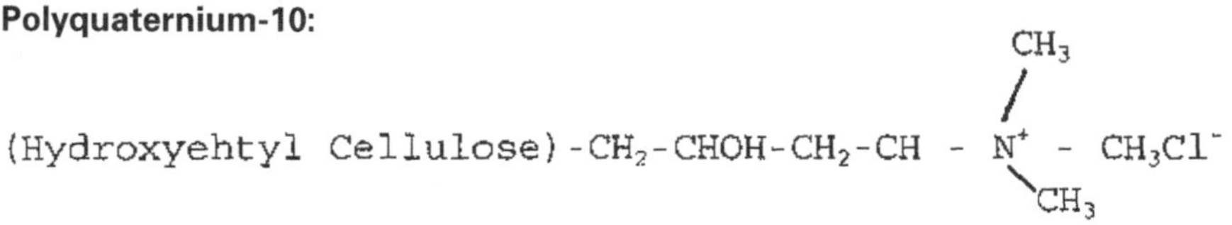
CH3
(Hydroxyehtyl Cellulose)-CH2-CHOH-CH2-CH - N+ - CH3Cl-
CH3

Polyquaternium-7:

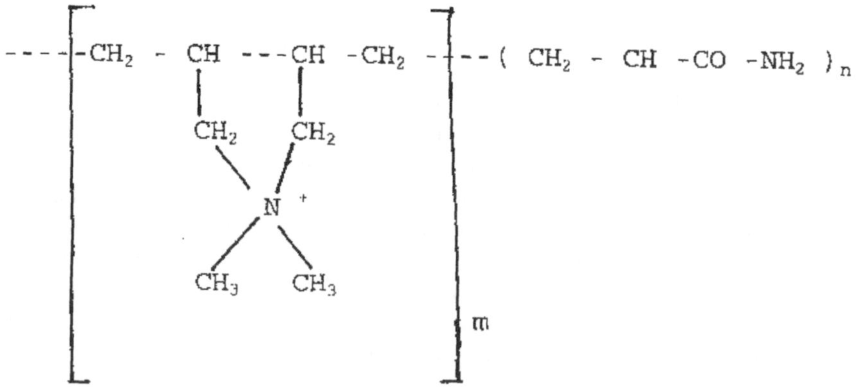
---CH2 - CH ---CH -CH2 ---(CH2 - CH -CO -NH2)n
CH2 CH2
N +
CH3 CH3
m

Polyquaternium-11:

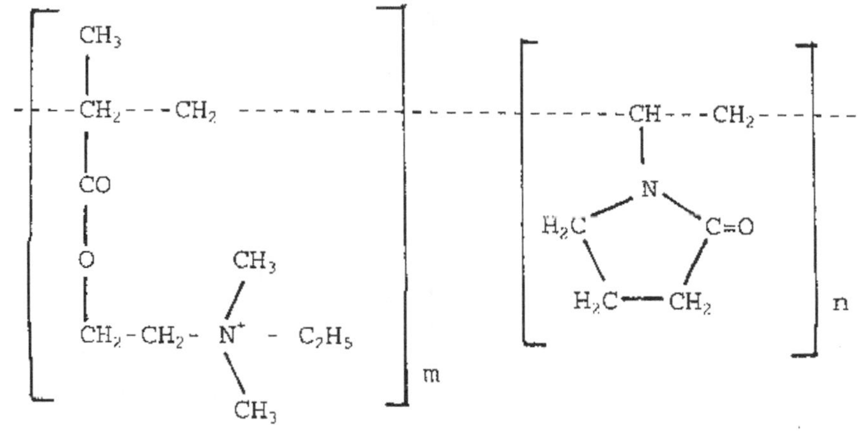

Guarhydroxypropyltrimethylammonium chloride:

$$\text{(Polysaccharide galactommannan)} - CHOH\text{-}CH_2\text{-}CH - \overset{\overset{\displaystyle CH_3}{|}}{\underset{\underset{\displaystyle CH_3}{|}}{N^+}} - CH_3Cl^-$$

Silicone Polymers. The silicone polymer most frequently used in two-in-one shampoos is dimethicone, while amodimethicone and dimethicone copolyol are also found occasionally. Dimethicone is an oil that is practically insoluble in water, making it a real challenge to use in shampoo formulations. The amodimethicone and dimethicone copolyol are modified dimethicone with organo-functional groups to increase the solubility and facilitate formulation [75]. The chemical structures of these three silicone polymers are as follows.

Dimethicone:

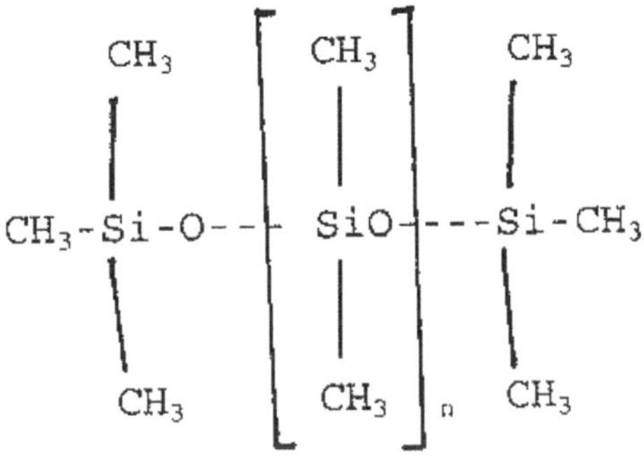

Amodimethicone:

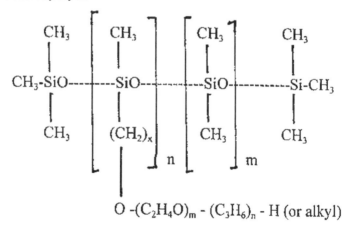

Dimethicone copolyol:

$$O -(C_2H_4O)_m - (C_3H_6)_n - H \text{ (or alkyl)}$$

4.3 Foam Boosters

Having a rich and copious foam in a shampoo is essential to consumer acceptance. Foam boosters are ingredients included in a shampoo to improve its lathering characteristics. Many of the anionic surfactants are good foamers, but the foams are mostly lacy and loose, especially in the presence of sebum or other oily materials. The function of foam boosters in two-in-one shampoos is particularly important when silicones are routinely used as conditioning agents. The two types foam booster most commonly used are discussed.

4.3.1 Fatty Acid Alkanolamides

The nonionic surfactants available as lauramide diethanolamine, cocamide diethanolamine, and cocamide monoethanolamine are fatty acid alkanolamides. These three surfactants alone at one point were believed to make up over 80% of the foam booster used for shampoos [73]. Of the three, the lauramide monoethanolamine is used more frequently because of the regulatory issue regarding the potential for N-nitrosamine formation from diethanolamines. The chemical structures of these three alkanolamides are as follows.

Lauramide diethethanolamine:

$$CH_3(CH_2)_{10}CON(CH_2CH_2OH)_2$$

Cocamidediethanol amine:

$$RCON(CH_2CH_2OH)_2$$

Cocamidemonoethanol amine:

$$RCONH-CH_2CH_2OH$$

where R is a coconut acid radical.

4.3.2 Betaines and Amine Oxides

Materials also found to be effective foam boosters for shampoos include betaines and amine oxides. Both are ionic surfactants that tend to display cationic characteristics under the pH values at which shampoos are normally formulated. The important betaine and amine oxides used in shampoos as foam boosters are cocamidopropyl betaine, cocamidopropyl hydroxysultaine, lauramine oxide, dihydroxyethyl C12–15 alkoxypropylamine oxide, and cocamidopropylamine oxide (see structures that follow).

Cocamidopropyl betaine:

$$R(CO)NH(CH_2)_3N^+(CH_3)_2CH_2OO^-$$

Cocamidopropyl hydroxysultaine:

$$R(CO)NH(CH_2)_3N^+(CH_3)_2CH_2CH(OH)CH_2SO_3$$

Lauramine oxide:

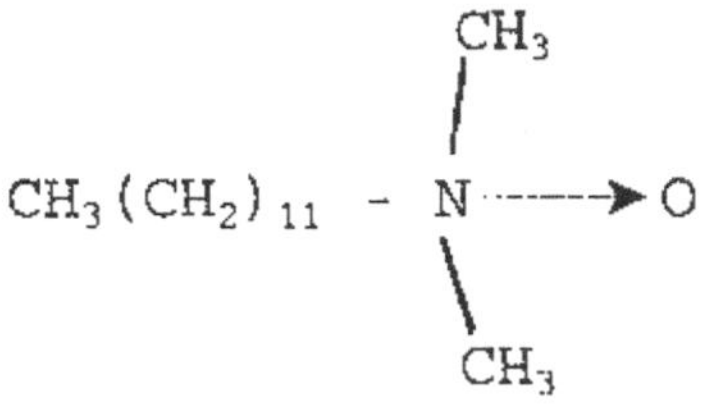

$$CH_3(CH_2)_{11} - \overset{\overset{\displaystyle CH_3}{|}}{\underset{\underset{\displaystyle CH_3}{\diagdown}}{N}} \cdots\!\!\longrightarrow O$$

Cocamine oxide:

$$R - \overset{\overset{\displaystyle CH_3}{|}}{\underset{\underset{\displaystyle CH_3}{|}}{N}} \longrightarrow O$$

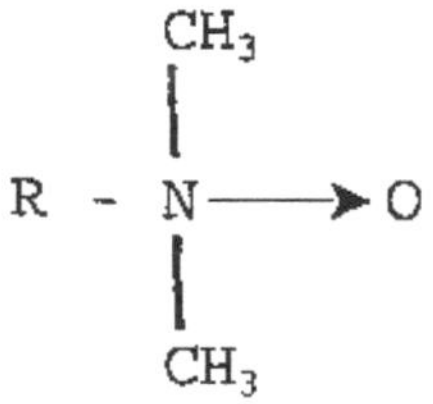

Dihydroxyethyl C$_{12\text{-}15}$ alkoxypropylamine oxide:

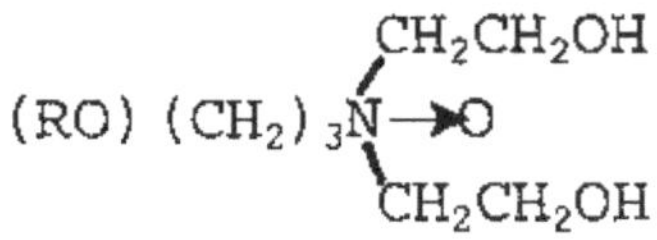

$$(RO)(CH_2)_3\overset{\diagup CH_2CH_2OH}{\underset{\diagdown CH_2CH_2OH}{N}}\!\!\!\!\longrightarrow O$$

where R is a coconut acid radical.

The uses of amine oxides have been somewhat restrained by the concern that some of them (such as lauramine oxide and stearamine oxide) are potential precursors of N-nitrosamine [76,77].

4.4 Preservatives

Effective preservatives for shampoos are essential to protect against microbial growth that could cause spoilage of the product, or more importantly, pose a health hazard to consumers. For two-in-one shampoos, the choice of a proper preservative system is even more critical because xof the incorporation of conditioning agents, such as silicone or hydrolyzed proteins, that are believed to support the growth and propagation of microorganisms, in particular the gram-negative family of *Pseudomonas* [78–80]. Formaldehyde used to be popular but has been largely replaced because of toxicological concerns. Other compounds that are found to be effective preservatives and are frequently used in shampoos [76,81] are methyl and propyl parahydroxy benzoates alone or in combination with imidazolidinyl urea, methylisothiazolinone, methyloldiethylhydantoin (DMDMH), methychloroisothiazolinone, and N-(3-chloroallyl)-hexaminium chloride (quaternium 15). The selection of a suitable preservative, however, must be customized for a specific shampoo formulation to achieve the proper trade-off between efficacy, safety, and compatibility [82–86].

5 CONCLUDING REMARKS

Consumer needs have been the main driving force behind the flurries of innovations and research activities in the evolution of the two-in-one conditioning shampoos. The formulation technology of these products has advanced considerably over the years, made possible by the discovery of the "dilution–deposition" phenomenon, as well as the utilization of silicone polymers. Nowadays, it is routine for an experienced formulator to put together a conditioning shampoo that would meet all the essential product and performance expectations. The key is to recognize the appropriate combinations of ingredients that will allow both the hair cleaning process and hair conditioning process to operate effectively. In theory, the principle of this technological approach can be applied to formulate other types of multifunctional shampoos: a shampoo that delivers temporary hair color, for example; or a shampoo that provides properties useful in the styling or setting of hair. It is not the technical feasibility that is in question. It is again the consumer needs and demands for such multifunctional products that determine the amounts of future innovations and research activities similar to those that were behind the two-in-one shampoos.

REFERENCES

1. Haati E. Scand J Clin Lab Invest 13:1 (1961).
2. Felger CB. J Soc Cosmet Chem 20:565 (1969).
3. Gloor M, Kionke M, Friederick HC. Arch Dermatol Res 251:317 (1975).
4. Breuer MM. J Soc Cosmet Chem 32:437 (1981).
5. Montagna W, ed. Advances in the Biology of the Skin, Vol 4. Oxford: Pergamon Press, 1963.
6. Eberhardt H, Arch Dermatol Forsch 251:155 (1974).
7. Leduc M, Maes D, Nadvornik JM, Reinstein JA, Turek BA, Vieu V. Studies on the regreasing of hair. Tenth Congress of the International Federation of Societies of Cosmetic Chemists, Melbourne, Australia, 1978.
8. Sanders HL, Lambert JM. J Am Oil Chem Soc 27:153 (1950).
9. Harry RG. Modern Cosmetology, 4th ed. London: Leonard Hill, 1955.
10. Adams NK. J Soc Dyers Color 53:121 (1937).
11. Stevenson DG. J Text Inst 44:T12 (1953).
12. Stevenson DG. J Text Inst 50:T548 (1959).
13. Preston WC. J Phys Chem 52:84 (1948).
14. Chan AF, Evans DF, Cussler EL. AICHE J 22:1006 (1976).
15. Schaewitz JA, Chan AF, Cussler EL, J Colloid Interface Sci 84:47 (1981).
16. Brash SV, Amoore JA. J Soc Cosmet Chem 18:31 (1967).

17. Heinz KL, Velder-Van der Ende, Cosmet Perfume 88:41 (1973).
18. Thompson D, Lemaster C, Allen R, J Soc Cosmet Chem 36:271 (1985).
19. Bore P, Goetz N, Gataud P, Tourenq L. Int J Cosmet Sci 4:39 (1982).
20. Wong M, Conklin E. Evaluation of cleansing action of shampoos. Annual Scientific
     Seminar of the Society of Cosmetic Chemists, Washington, DC, May 1976.
21. Surfactant Encyclopedia. Cosmet Toiletries 104:67 (February 1989).
22. Verdicchio R, Walts J. US Patent 3,950,417 (1976).
23. Blake-Haskins JC, Scala D, Rhein LD, Robbins CR. J Soc Cosmet Chem 37:199
     (1986).
24. Hunting LL. Cosmet Toiletries 100:58 (March 1974).
25. Alexander P. Cosmet Perfume 90:21 (July 1975).
26. Gerstein T. Cosmet Toileteries 93:15 (February 1978).
27. Tolgyesi E. Breask AF, Cosmet Toiletries 96:57 (July 1981).
28. Hunting ALL. Cosmet Toiletries 103:73 (March 1988).
29. Colgate Palmolive. US Patent 3,697,452 (1972).
30. Colgate Palmolive. US Patent 3,810,478 (1974).
31. Procter & Gamble. US Patent 3,313,734 (1967).
32. National Starch. US Patent 4,009265 (1977).
33. American Cyanamid. US Patent 4,001,394 (1977).
34. Colgate Palmolive. US Patent 3,496,110 (1970).
35. Scott V, Robbins CR, Barnhurst JD. J Soc Cosmet Chem 20:135 (1969).
36. Finkelstein P, Laden K. The mechanism of conditioning of hair with alkyl quaternary
     ammonium compounds. Proceedings of the Fourth International Wool Textile
     Research Conference, Part I, 1971.
37. Hilfer H. Drug Cosmet Ind 73:766 (1953).
38. Doubleday C. Soap Perfum Cosmet 76:263 (1953).
39. Lewis WF. Soap Perfum Cosmet 28:642 (1955).
40. Cosmet Toiletries 103:113 (March 1988).
41. Goddard ED, Hannan RB. J. Colloid Interface Science 55(1):73 (1976).
42. Tomlinson E, Davis SS, Mukhayer GI. In: KL Mittal, ed. Solution Chemistry of Sur-
     factants, Vol 1. New York: Plenum Press, 1979, p 3.
43. Lucassen-Reynders EH, Lucassen J, Giles D. J Colloid Interface Sci 81:150 (1981).
44. Bourrel M, Bernard D, Graciaa A. Tenside Deterg 21(6):311 (1984).
45. Mehreteab A, Loprest FJ. J Colloid Interface Sci 125:602 (1988).
46. Goddard ED. J Soc Cosmet Chem 41:23 (1990).
47. Warner Lambert. US Patent 3,816,616 (1974).
48. L'Oréal. British Patent 1,416,454 (1975).
49. L'Oréal. US Patent 4,048,301 (1977).
50. Beecham. British Patent. 1,540,384 (1979).
51. Shiseido Co. US Patent 4,919,846 (1990).
52. Cosmet Toiletries 103:114 (March 1988).
53. Cosmet Toiletries 106:84 (April 1991).
54. Oven MJ. CHEMTECH pp 288 (May 1981).
55. Starch ME. Drug Cosmet Ind 134:38 (June 1988).
56. US Patent 2,826,551 (1958).
57. British Patent 849,433 (1960).

58. Lever Brothers. US Patent 3,946,500 (1976).
59. Lever Brothers. US Patent 4,364,837 (1982).
60. Kao Corp. US Patent 4,479,893 (1984).
61. Procter & Gamble. US Patent 4,728,457 (1988).
62. Procter & Gamble. US Patent 4,788,006 (1988).
63. Halloran DJ, Household Pers Prod Ind 28:60 (November 1991).
64. Branna T, Household Pers Prod Ind 28:43 (November 1991).
65. Berthiaume MD, Merifield JH, Ricco DA. J Soc. Cosmet Chem 46:231 (1995).
66. Kao Corp. British Patent 2,255,101 (1993).
67. Goze J. US Patent 5,015,415 (1993).
68. Calgon. EP Patent Application 521,666 (1992).
69. Yahagi K. J Soc Cosmet Chem 43:275 (1992).
70. Hallogran DJ. Cosmet Chem Spec 68:22 (1992).
71. Sajic B, Shapiro I. Cosmet Toiletrics 107:103 (May 1992).
72. Caelles J, Comelles F, Leal JS, Parra JL, Anguera S. Cosmet Toileteries 109:49 (April 1991).
73. Fox C. Cosmet Toiletries 103:25 (March 1988).
74. Cotrell PL. Cosmet Technol 27 (August 1982).
75. Wendal SR, DeSapio AJ. Cosmet Toiletries 98:103 (May 1983).
76. Wenninger JA. Household Pers Prod Ind 21(2) (February 1984).
77. Dickinson J. Cosmet Technol 3(7) (July 1981).
78. Yablonski JI, Goldman CI. Cosmet Perfum 90:45 (1975).
79. Bean HS, Heman-Ackah SM, Thomas J. J Soc Cosmet Chem 16:15 (1965).
80. Bryce DM, Smart R. J Soc Cosmet Chem 16:187 (1965).
81. Decker RL, Wenninger RL, Cosmet Toiletries 102:21 (December 1987).
82. Croshaw B. J Soc Cosmet Chem 28:3 (1977).
83. Moral J. Cosmet Toiletries 107:65 (1992).
84. Corbett RJ. Parfum Kosmet 73:22 (1992).
85. Doorne HV. Parfum Kosmet 73:84 (1992).
86. Dhsw A. Soaps Cosmet Chem Spec 70:32 (May 1994).

5

Aspects of Multifunctionality in Skin Care Products

Johann W. Wiechers
Uniqema, Gouda, The Netherlands

1 INTRODUCTION

The numerous examples of multifunctional personal care products in today's marketplace clearly illustrate the relevance of the concept of multifunctionality to modern cosmetic science. Effects, efficacies, and performances that were never considered to be associated are now being combined—for instance: color and moisture, UV blocking and suppleness. In theory, the number of combinations of efficacies is infinite. On paper, multifunctionality can be easily invented, but technically, it may be extremely difficult to find the chemicals that allow the cosmetic scientist to achieve these demanding requests of consumers and marketers.

For about a decade, the cosmetic industry has been looking at Nature to provide the chemistry that could deliver all these miraculous effects in a single molecule. This type of multifunctionality can be referred to as the "one-in-more" approach, since *one* ingredient has to be active *in more* than one functionality. But as cosmetic chemists strive for a much wider range of multifunctionality than existed a decade ago, it is realized that not every possible combination of two (or even more) functionalities can be delivered within a single molecule.

In this chapter, the focus will be on the feasibility of achieving multifunctionality via the "one-in-more" approach (i.e., within single molecules), as well as on achieving this by mixing individual ingredients that excel in a single specific performance. This latter method can be called the "more-in-one" approach, as *more* ingredients with distinctive efficacies are combined *in one* formulation to achieve a multifunctional cosmetic product.

Whereas some types of functionality easily go together, others seem to exclude each other. But before such a discussion can start, it is necessary to establish a definition of "functionality," for there are different meanings of this word, all equally correct. In this chapter, the functionality of a personal care ingredient is any function that this ingredient may have. This refers to individual ingredients, not final cosmetic formulations. This functionality of the ingredient can range from acting as a preservative to an emulsifier (a means to microbiologically or physically stabilize a formulation, respectively) to acting as a moisturizer or an emollient (which are means to positively influence the hydration level or the skin feel of a formulation, respectively). In this chapter, the focus will be on the latter types of functionality, namely, skin moisturization, skin elasticity, and skin feel.

For some time now, I have been measuring the relative performance of nonformulated personal care ingredients in skin moisturization, skin elasticity, and skin substantivity, as well as their sensory characteristics. A first observation was that not all personal care ingredients exert the same degree of efficacy toward these functionalities. When they were measured relative to a negative and a positive control, representing 0 and 100% performance, respectively, the ingredients could be subdivided into three groups with a low (< 30%), medium (30–70%), and high performance (> 70%). For example, Figs. 1 and 2 rank the relative moisturization and elasticity performance of a large group of personal care ingredients from low to high. Each bar represents a product, and products under the same horizontal arrow are not statistically significantly different from each other at the $p = 0.05$ level. Experimental details can be found elsewhere [1,2]. But when the performances in the various functionalities were plotted against each other, it was discovered that certain emollients were excellent in providing one functionality but poor in another, whereas for other nonformulated ingredients, the situation might be the other way round [2]. This is depicted in Fig. 3, where the relative elasticity performance of personal care ingredients is plotted as a function of their relative moisturization performance. Figure 3 shows two groups of chemicals, a series of ingredients with a low skin elasticity performance but a wide range of moisturization performances, and a series with a low moisturization performance but a wide range of skin elasticity performances. In other words, there were no ingredients that had a high performance in both moisturization and elasticity. None of these personal care ingredients had "one-in-more" potential. To create such a multifunctional product, the best moisturizing ingredient (which is poor in skin elastic-

Relative Performance (%)

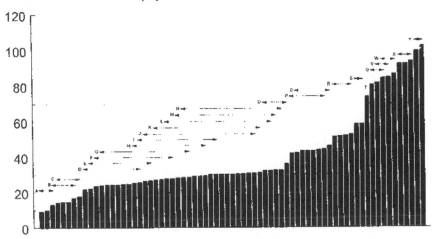

FIGURE 1   Ranking of personal care ingredient products by their skin moisturization performance at 6 hours, relative to glycerin-treated skin (100%) and untreated skin (0%).

Relative Performance (%)

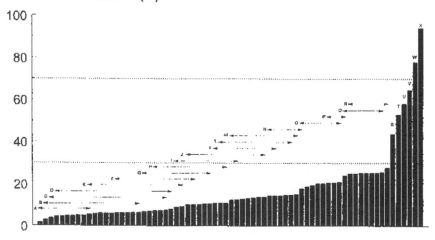

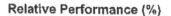

FIGURE 2   Ranking of personal care ingredient products by their skin elasticity performance at 6 hours, relative to water-treated skin for 30 minutes (100%) and untreated skin (0%).

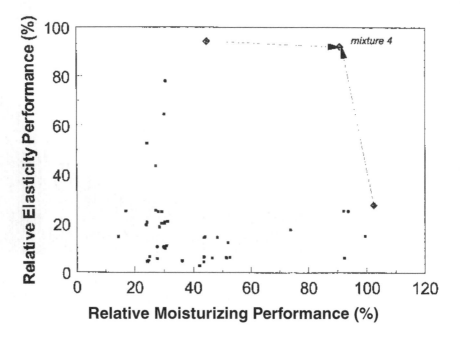

FIGURE 3   Relationship between moisturizing and plasticizing performance of personal care ingredients as well as an equimolar mixture of a good moisturizer and a good plasticizer (mixture 4).

ity) and the best elasticity-providing ingredient (which is poor in skin moisturization) were combined. The efficacy of this multifunctional mixture, mixture 4, is also indicated in Fig. 3 at the point where the two arrows meet. This mixture demonstrated a high performance in both functionalities, an effect that could not be obtained with any of the single ingredients.

A legitimate question, however, is this: Why did we not obtain the average effect of both mixture components in the mixture? After all, seen from the point of view of skin moisturization, a highly effective moisturizer was mixed with an ingredient of only low performance. As a consequence, a merely average skin moisturization and skin elasticity performance of the mixture might have been expected. This is an example of synergy between cosmetic ingredients, which must, of course, exist. After all, most cosmetic formulations are mixtures of many ingredients, and without the existence of such synergies, every formulation would have been roughly the same (i.e., average) with respect to its functionalities. Since this is not the case, synergies and antagonistic effects must exist, but they have never been systematically investigated.

This chapter describes the multifunctionality of mixtures of ingredients that individually excel in a certain skin functionality. Both synergistic and antagonistic effects have been observed. Although the research into this subject is ongoing and full explanations for the occurrence of such synergies cannot yet be given, enough interesting examples are already available to justify this chapter in a book called *Multifunctional Cosmetics.*

2 MEASURING RELATIVE PERFORMANCE

Two types of measurement were performed by using the Relative Performance technique [1,3]. Skin moisturization and skin elasticity were measured following application of emollients by means of noninvasive skin bioengineering instruments. Negative and positive control products were always included that represented 0% and 100% performance, respectively. The reference products, however, were different for skin moisturization and skin elasticity.

In a second set of studies, completely independent of the instrumental studies, highly trained human panels were used as the measuring instrument when the skin sensory characteristics of nonformulated personal care ingredients were assessed. The performance of ingredients toward the various sensory attributes was also measured on a 100-point scale, which is characterized by various reference samples. As with the relative performance scales used for skin moisturization and skin elasticity, the sensory scales use different references depending on the attribute under study.

2.1 Instrumental Measurements

Skin moisturization was assessed via measurement of the capacitance of the superficial layers of the stratum corneum. The Corneometer CM820 (Courage & Khazaka, Cologne, Germany) measures the time needed to load the plates of a capacitor placed on the skin surface. The amount of charge that this capacitor can carry depends on the dielectric constant of the medium between its plates. The Corneometer has been constructed in such a way that this medium between the plates is the stratum corneum and to a lesser extent, when placed on the skin, the viable epidermis and dermis. The dielectric constant of most personal care ingredients, certainly the more lipophilic emollients, is quite low and on the order of 2–3 [4]. It increases with the polarity and dipole moment within a molecule. Water has an extremely high dielectric constant at 20°C, about 80. Extremely dry skin does not contain large quantities of water and, as a consequence, its dielectric constant is quite low. As we go from dry to normal skin, the quantity of water in the skin increases, and so does the dielectric constant and therefore the time needed to load the plates of the capacitor. The Corneometer does not measure the absolute quantity of water in the skin but a derived parameter that is in line with the absolute water content. Care should be taken with the interpretation of results of chemicals that have a reasonable high dielectric constants, such as ethanol ($\varepsilon =$ 24.3 at 25°C) and glycerin ($\varepsilon = 42.5$ at 25°C) [5]. An increased value with these chemicals does not necessarily mean increased hydration; it could just be the uptake of the product in the skin itself.

We have always used glycerin as the positive control in our experiments, and have therefore asked whether we were measuring changes in the skin's water content or just the uptake of glycerin into the skin. An easy way to check this is to assess the value the Corneometer reaches when a tissue soaked with the product is measured. The higher the dielectric constant of the product or the ingredient, the higher the value of the Corneometer will be. But if the same product applied to the skin is—after a couple of hours—yielding values significantly higher than that achieved on the soaked tissue, one knows that one is also measuring water, although some contribution of the product itself can never be excluded. We measured values around 115 for skin to which glycerin had been applied for 6 hours using the Corneometer CM820 [1], and values around 60 for filter papers soaked with the same glycerin.

All personal care ingredients or mixtures thereof were applied for 6 hours on skin of healthy volunteers who gave their written, informed consent. Upon removal of the remaining product, measurements were taken on the volar aspect of the left forearm after acclimatization for at least 30 minutes in a temperature-controlled room (21 ± 0.5°C) at a relative humidity of $45 \pm 5\%$. All measurements were taken in triplicate, and each ingredient or mixture was tested on 20 subjects of either sex.

Skin elasticity was measured by means of a Dermal Torque Meter (DTM) (Dia-Stron, Andover, Hampshire, U.K.). This equipment consists of two concentric rings of which the inner rotates relative to a static outer ring with a given torque. Both rings are attached to the skin by means of double-sided sticky tape. The more elastic skin is, the greater the angle of immediate deformation will be after a short fixed period of time following application of the torque. Because the rings are concentric, forces are applied in two dimensions of an xy plane, whereas the gap width between the rings determines the depth of measurement. If the gap is wide (> 2 mm), the applied forces can penetrate deeply into the skin and the measured angle is predominantly determined by the deeper skin layers such as the dermal layers. As the gap width narrows, the influence of the deeper layers is reduced. At a gap width of 1 mm, the influence of the dermal component can almost be ignored relative to that of the stratum corneum [6]. This clearly indicates that the DTM is actually measuring in an xyz space. Recent developments in skin elasticity indicate that the elasticity is dependent on the direction of the fibroblasts in the skin and therefore dependent on the direction in which it is measured [7].

In our skin elasticity experiments using the DTM with a gap width of only 1 mm, we measured the U_E, the immediate elastic deformation of the skin due to the application of the torque. This is the angle of deformation after 50 ms relative to the situation before applying the strain. The value of U_E depends on the thickness of the skin [8], and one should therefore measure this by means of, for instance, ultrasound. However, because the performance of each ingredient or mixture thereof was measured relative to a positive and negative control on the same individual at the same time on nearby sites (and thus with approximately the same stratum corneum thickness), it is no longer necessary to measure this variable separately. Single measurements were taken on the back of volunteers, 6 hours after product application and following removal of the dose. As slight amounts of remaining product could potentially result in insufficient adherence of the double-sided sticky tape, subsequently yielding an artificially high value for U_E, we checked for the presence of any remaining product following removal of the dose by means of a Sebumeter (Courage & Khazaka). A single measurement was taken. For the rest, the experimental conditions were identical to those described for moisturisation above.

Relative performance values (RP) were calculated according to the formula:

$$RP \; (\%) = \frac{\text{test} - NC}{PC - NC} \; 100\% \tag{5.1}$$

for both moisturization and elasticity. In this formula, test, PC, and NC are the values obtained for the Corneometer or Dermal Torque Meter for the test product (single ingredient or mixture), positive control and negative control, respectively. The positive controls for skin moisturization and skin elasticity were glycerin and water, respectively, applied for 30 minutes under occlusion. Control values were always measured at the same time as the test products (6 h), except for the positive control for elasticity, which was only taken at 30 minutes.

2.2 Sensory Measurements

Trained panels applied set quantities of nonformulated personal care ingredients to their skin (50 µL) and judged the performance of each ingredient with respect to 20 predefined attributes. These attributes were subdivided with regards to the time of observation: pickup, rubout, and afterfeel immediately after product application as well as after 20 minutes. The panel consisted of 11 highly trained women. Single ingredients or mixtures thereof were evaluated only once in separate studies, but some single ingredients were remeasured to check for consistency. No statistically significant differences were found between the first and second evaluation of the same product for any of the 20 attributes. This allowed the two data sets to be merged into one single data set.

Sensory studies tend to yield a tremendous amount of data, and it is often difficult to differentiate between all the effects. After all, one is working in a 20-dimensional space when dealing with 20 attributes. To make sense of it all, principal component analysis (PCA) has been demonstrated to be a useful statistical technique. This method identifies linear correlations in the data set and combines effects that are highly correlated. In doing so, it reduces the number of dimensions, often significantly, but the new composite dimensions have become meaningless. More detail on the construction and meaning of PCA in skin sensory research is given in the literature [9,10].

Figure 4 shows a PCA loading plot of all the attributes after completion of a single-ingredient study [11]. In short, when two vectors are close together, the effects they represent are highly correlated (but for reasons of clarity, one does not plot the vectors, and the position of the attribute in a diagram is therefore important). For instance, when the greasiness that is perceived immediately after product application (GRS___) increases, the greasiness after 20 minutes (GRS___20)

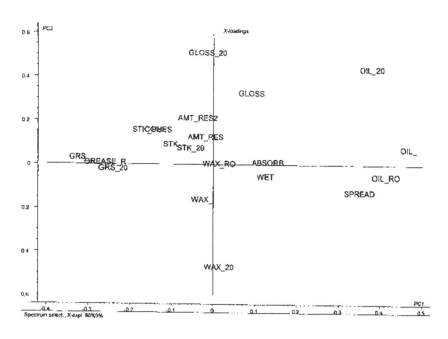

FIGURE 4 Principal component analysis loading plot of the attributes used in the sensory study investigating nonformulated personal care ingredients. Attributes that are positioned together are highly positively correlated, whereas those mirrored in the origin are highly negatively correlated. Attributes at an angle of about 90° are not correlated.

also increases. These two attributes are therefore positioned closely together in Fig. 4. Likewise, when two attributes are inversely correlated—as for instance, oiliness (OIL___) and greasiness (GRS___)—their positions are mirrored in the origin of the PCA plot.

From such a PCA loading plot as Fig. 4, one can immediately identify which skin efficacies cannot be combined in one product. It is anticipated that it will be almost impossible to create a mixture that has a high score for 20 minutes after-feel on both wax (WAX___20) and gloss (GLOSS___20) because these efficacies are mirrored in the origin of the PCA loading plot and thus inversely correlated. If the value of WAX___20 increases, that of GLOSS___20 decreases, and vice versa. Oiliness and greasiness also do not easily go together. However, it should always be realized that this is only true within the set of products studied, although our data set with its 59 personal care ingredients may be considered to be quite comprehensive.

3 CRITERIA FOR SELECTING SINGLE INGREDIENTS FOR MIXTURES

When one is aiming to make a multifunctional mixture from two ingredients, both of which excel in another property, it is most likely that one also will make a mixture of a high performer and a medium or low performer *within* these two properties. In the example of the mixture shown in Fig. 3, where a good moisturizer was mixed with a good skin elasticity provider, a good moisturizer was also mixed with a poor moisturizer and a poor elasticity provider with a high-performance elasticity provider. One should therefore also consider separately the single efficacies that are combined in the multifunctional mixture. To investigate the influence of mixing within a single efficacy, we made all possible six combinations of poor, medium, and high efficacy: poor/poor, poor/medium, poor/high, medium/medium, medium/high, and high/high. Because of the high number of skin functionalities measured (moisturization, elasticity, and the 20 sensory attributes), this could not be done for all skin efficacies. We therefore decided to concentrate on moisturization, elasticity, and only a few relevant sensory attributes, predominantly relating to gloss and greasiness.

For sensory properties, we tested 18 mixtures. For skin moisturization and elasticity, we tested 10 mixtures, some of which were also tested for their sensory properties. In these experiments, we also incorporated a few single ingredients to check the repeatability of the instrumental or sensory test. Only when this is the case can one merge the data from previously obtained single ingredients with the data of the newly obtained mixtures. All mixtures were made as 50:50 mixtures on a molar ratio basis; that is, the number of molecules was the same for each ingredient. The reason for this, instead of simply mixing 50:50 by weight or volume, was to facilitate prediction of the average performance assuming ideal behavior. The mixtures were tested under exactly the same conditions as the single ingredients.

4   RESULTS OF INSTRUMENTAL AND SENSORY MIXTURE STUDIES

Some typical results of the mixture study for skin moisturization and elasticity are shown in Fig. 5, which like Fig. 3 shows two functionalities in one graph (elasticity performance of single ingredients, as well as some mixtures as a function of their moisturization potential) of both ingredients and the mixture. Such a graph allows a quick overview of how the mixture performs relative to the single ingredients that make up the mixture. For this reason, this type of plot is called a multifunctionality plot.

However, this type of graphical display makes it very difficult to obtain an overview of synergies or antagonistic effects within a single functionality, and therefore one also shows the same data in another format. The composition of mixtures of two ingredients can be represented by the position on a line of which the

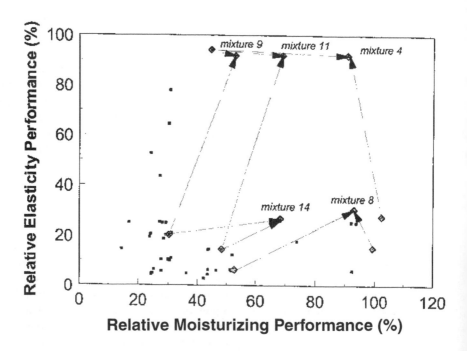

FIGURE 5   Multifunctionality plot of some more representative, equimolar mixtures (mixtures 8, 9, 11, and 14).

Moisturization

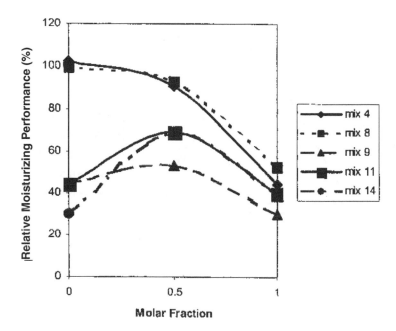

FIGURE 6   Single functionality plot of the moisturization performance of the same mixtures shown in Fig. 5.

extremes represent the pure ingredients. If one allows different products to be represented at either end, more than one mixture can be displayed in the same graph. The same mixtures shown in Fig. 5 are illustrated in Figs. 6 (moisturization) and 7 (elasticity), respectively. These plots are called single functionality plots because they allow quick identification of synergy within a single functionality.

For reasons of simplicity, the results from the skin sensory mixture study are shown only as single functionality plots in Figs. 8 and 9, similar to Figs. 6 and 7. Only a few characteristic examples are shown, illustrating the various types of interaction that are possible.

5   DISCUSSION

Classical skin bioengineering techniques and sensory methods were used to test nonformulated personal care ingredients for their relative performance on skin moisturization and skin elasticity as well as for their skin sensory characteristics. In a subsequent series of experiments, mixtures of some of these ingredients were

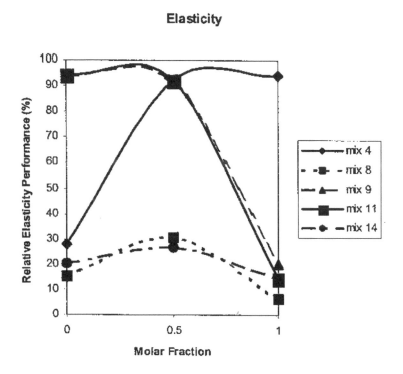

FIGURE 7 Single functionality plot of the elasticity performance of the same mixtures shown in Fig. 5.

prepared to study the interaction between individual chemicals. Two ways of studying the data could be distinguished: one can look at multifunctionality (i.e., both functionalities at the same time) or at single functionality (i.e., within one functionality).

When mixtures are made of two ingredients that have different degrees of performance on a given functionality, three outcomes are possible. First, the mixture might have the average performance of the two individual ingredients that make up the mixture. In such a case, the mixture is demonstrating linear behavior, which means that its effect can be predicted from that of the individual ingredients according to the molar fractions of each of its components, according to the formula:

$$\text{Efficacy mixture} = X_1 P_1 + X_2 P_2 \tag{5.2}$$

where X_1 and X_2 are the molar fractions of ingredient 1 and 2, respectively, and P_1 and P_2 their respective skin performances. The efficacy of such a mixture is there-

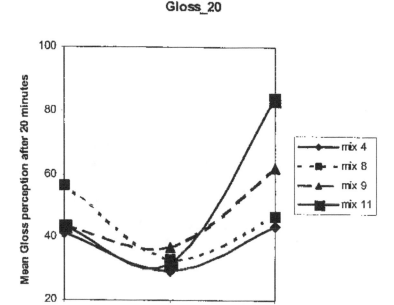

FIGURE 8 Single functionality plot of the skin sensory performance (gloss perception 20 min after application) of the same mixtures shown in Fig. 5.

fore an arithmetic mean of the individual performances. A poor example of this behavior is mixture 8 in Fig. 9. It is only a poor example, because the line is not perfectly straight.

Second, the performance of the mixture might be greater than the arithmetic mean and thus show a synergistic effect, according to the formula:

$$\text{Efficacy mixture} > X_1P_1 + X_2P_2 \tag{5.3}$$

This is often called synergy, but that is not necessarily a valid description because it depends on the desired effect. For moisturization, Eq. (5.3) would be said to reflect synergy, whereas for sensory attributes like greasiness and gloss (neither of which is desired), performance according to Eq. (5.3) would be considered to be antagonistic. It is even impossible to generalize for performances. For example, whereas skin gloss is undesired, hair gloss is highly desired. The definition of synergy therefore varies from property to property. Clear examples of synergy are given in Fig. 6, where all mixtures yield more moisturization than the arithmetic means of their individual components. Mixtures 4, 8, and 9 in Fig. 7 are beautiful

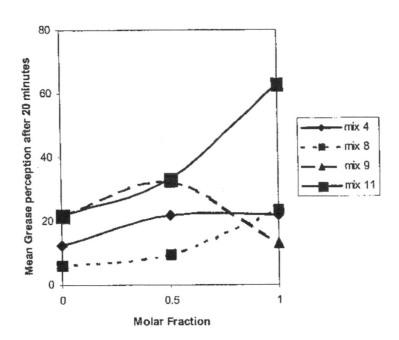

FIGURE 9 Single functionality plot of the skin sensory performance (grease perception 20 min after application) of the same mixtures as shown in Fig. 5.

examples of synergy in skin elasticity. Although all lines are going down in Fig. 8, the effect is still called synergy, since glossiness of skin is not desired.

Third, the performance of the mixture can be smaller than the arithmetic mean of the individual components according to the formula:

$$\text{Efficacy mixture} < X_1 P_1 + X_2 P_2 \tag{5.4}$$

which would be seen to be an antagonistic effect in most cases. An example of antagonism is mixture 9 in Fig. 9: although the line is going up, greasiness is not sought after, and because the mixture yields more greasiness than either single ingredient, it is therefore an example of antagonism.

Because of the possible confusion regarding synergy and antagonism depending on the desirability of the effect, the concept of superfunctionality should be introduced. Superfunctionality is here defined as an interaction between two ingredients making the mixture more desirable in one functionality (i.e., better) than the performance of the individual ingredients making up the mixture.

Superfunctionality is therefore more than just performance above the arithmetic mean. Whether this occurs can be seen in single-functionality plots such as Figs. 6–9. Examples of superfunctionality are mixtures 9, 11, and 14 in skin moisturization (Fig. 6), 8 and 14 in skin elasticity (Fig. 7), and all mixtures in glossiness after 20 minutes (Fig. 8). Although a synergistic effect is seen for mixture 8 in greasiness (Fig. 9), none of the mixtures is superfunctional because the performance of the mixtures never exceeds that of the individual components.

If superfunctionality happens in two functionalities at the same time (e.g., in mixture 14 in Fig. 5), this is called a supermultifunctional mixture. The existence of supermultifunctionality can be best observed in multifunctionality plots, such as Figs. 3 and 5.

In the discussion of the composition of multifunctional mixtures, it was noted that the two ingredients that make up this mixture are often completely different in their chemical composition, which makes perfect sense. For instance, for the more biological effects like moisturization and elasticity, molecules with similar structures are more likely to work by a similar mechanism than structures that are completely different. Although the molecular basis for skin moisturization is still unclear [2], one might, for instance, anticipate the combination of a humectant and an occluding personal care ingredient to be more effective than a mixture of two humectants or two occluding agents. Actually, for performances based more on physical chemistry such as occlusion and gloss, the formation of regular molecular arrangements in the film covering the skin is required to observe such effects. By inserting chemicals with more or less the same chemical structure, such molecular arrangements may still be formed, albeit slightly less perfectly. However, when the two ingredients in the mixture have completely different chemical structures, such regular molecular arrangements often cannot be made and properties like gloss will be lost, as can be seen in Fig. 8.

6   CONCLUSION

Cosmetics are no longer just fulfilling the needs of the more vain creatures among us. Current cosmetics actually have to work, and this requirement is only increasing. A single type of efficacy is often no longer sufficient, and the cosmetic industry has therefore sought for multifunctional cosmetics. Initially, this has solely been in the form of incorporating an active ingredient that had at least two different types of activity. However, the needs of today's consumer for multifunctionality are developing faster than the cosmetic industry can identify new active ingredients that can deliver these forms of multifunctionality. This chapter therefore describes another form of multifunctionality. Rather than obtaining this from a single ingredient, it describes the combination of two effective ingredients, each of which excels in a single specific property. It was possible to create multifunctional mixtures that delivered such effects. Because high-performing ingredients are mixed with less well performing chemicals, this approach requires synergistic effects between ingredients. Examples of synergistic and antagonistic combinations of ingredients as well as ideal behavior (the arithmetic mean performance of the two individual components of a mixture) were provided. It was observed that ingredients with different chemical structures had a higher probability of yielding synergy than ingredients similar in chemical structure.

REFERENCES

1. Wiechers JW. A supplier's contribution to performance testing of personal care ingredients. SOFW 123:981–990 (1997).
2. Wiechers JW, Barlow A. Skin moisturisation and elasticity originate from at least two different mechanisms. Int J Cosmet Sci 21:425–435 (1999).
3. Wiechers JW. Relative performance testing: Introducing a tool to facilitate cosmetic ingredient selection. Cosmet Toiletries 112(9):79–84 (1997).
4. Barel AO, Clarys P. In vitro calibration of the capacitance method (Corneometer CM825) for the evaluation of the hydration state of the skin. Active Ingredients, Conference Proceedings 1997, Verlag für chemische Industrie, Augsburg Germany, pp 21–38.
5. Weast RC, Astle MJ, eds. Handbook of Chemistry and Physics, 60th ed. Boca Raton, FL: CRC Press, 1979, pp E55–E61.
6. De Rigal J, Lévêque J-L. In-vivo measurement of the stratum corneum elasticity. Bioeng Skin, 1:13–23 (1985).
7. Vexler A, Polyansky I, Gorodetsky R. Evaluation of skin viscoelasticity and anisotropy by measurement of speed of shear wave propagation with viscoelastic analyzer (VESA). J Invest Dermatol 45:893–900 (1999).
8. Escoffier C, De Rigal J, Rochefort A, Vasselet R, Lévêque J-L, Agache PG. Age-related mechanical properties of human skin: An in-vivo study. J Invest Dermatol 93:353–357 (1989).
9. Wortel VAL, Wiechers JW. Skin sensory performance of individual personal care ingredients and marketed personal care products. Food Qual Preference 11:121–127 (2000).
10. Wiechers JW, Wortel VAL. Making sense of sensory data. Cosmet Toiletries 115(3):37–45 (2000).
11. Wiechers JW, Wortel VAL. Bridging the language gap between cosmetic formulators and consumers. Cosmet Toiletries 115(5):33–41 (2000).

6

Multifunctional Nail Care Products

Francis Busch

ProStrong, Inc., Oakville, Connecticut, U.S.A.

Nail care products offer an important opportunity to produce more than one function in the same product. Some nail care products by their very nature provide more than one function, for example, nail polish affords decoration and protection.

This chapter explores the opportunity for additional multifunctional nail cosmetics by first reviewing the structure and chemistry of a normal nail and then comparing the needs of this structure with the opportunity presented in each nail care product category. Since the basic structure of the nail is made up of cells that are fully keratinized, opportunities are explored to improve the durability of the nail by utilizing elements of nail chemistry amenable to treatment by cosmetic ingredients. In most cases, since one element of most nail cosmetics is either decorative or totally utilitarian, a multifunctional product will result. Examples of existing products that provide novel multifunctionality will be given when useful.

1 STRUCTURAL ELEMENTS OF THE HUMAN FINGERNAIL

Because the chemistry and physical properties of the nail are very complex, it is helpful to understand some of the elements of nail structure before formulating nail care products. As can be seen from a simplified schematic (Fig. 1), the nail consists of three major layers. While the cells that eventually form the top two lay-

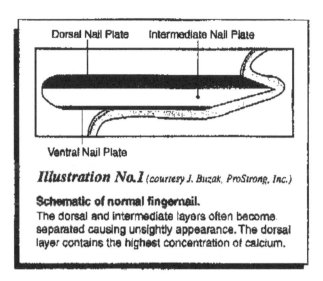

Illustration No.1 (courtesy J. Buzak, ProStrong, Inc.)

Schematic of normal fingernail.
The dorsal and intermediate layers often become
separated causing unsightly appearance. The dorsal
layer contains the highest concentration of calcium.

FIGURE 1   Schematic of normal fingernail. The dorsal and intermediate layers often become separated causing unsightly appearance. The dorsal layer contains the highest concentration of calcium. (Courtesy of J. Buzak, ProStrong, Inc.)

ers of nail are generated in the nail matrix and have much in common, important differences in cell chemistry and physical properties have been identified which explain differences in the texture of the respective layers [1]. The upper dorsal layer is the hardest of the three and not coincidentally contains the highest level of calcium [1]. This elevated level of calcium has in the last several years presented an important opportunity to improve the strength of the nail. Products based on this chemistry will be discussed in Sec. 2 on nail strengtheners and Sec. 5 on nail enamel. The middle layer, called the intermediate nail plate, is nearly twice as thick as the upper dorsal layer, and its cells are not as densely packed as in the dorsal layer. The lowest layer is called the ventral nail plate and is very thin: a mere one or two cell layers thick. This layer is generally not amenable to cosmetic treatment. The chemistry of each layer varies, and this variance contributes at least in part to the structural differences of the nail. Chemically the nail is a hard keratin and contains various metals in small amounts. The three-layered nail plate is made up of flattened cells compacted into the protective shield covering the tips of our fingers. While the difference in texture observed between the three layers is not clearly understood, it likely results from differences in the degree of cell flattening as the three layers form, differences in calcium content, and formation of disulfide linkages among the amino acids making up the basic keratin structure.

The nail matrix producing the top two layers of nail plate does not lie directly beneath the nail but prior to the nail just below the lunula (the half-moon-shaped surface as the nail begins). The thin ventral nail plate is thought to be formed directly from the nail bed, but some of the cells could be produced from the nail matrix. All the cells making up the dorsal and intermediate nail plates are flattened and dehydrated. Since they are not living cells, the concept of nail nutrition from a topically applied cosmetic is irrational. This does not mean that the nonliving material making up the principal parts of the nail cannot be treated, but it is important to remember that you are working with an inanimate material. When formulating nail products, I first try to visualize things that could affect a small piece of hard, semirigid plastic formed in layers.

The cosmetic chemist is primarily interested in the dorsal layer of the nail, the cuticle and the skin adjacent to the sides of the nail. This latter skin can become thick and quite irritated. Once this adjacent tissue becomes broken (hangnails, etc.), it is not easily treated with typical hand creams and presents to the formulator an opportunity to develop a multifunctional cuticle product that will provide badly needed help.

Another opportunity for the cosmetic chemist lies in the fact that the layers of the nail can become separated. We formulators hear complaints daily about peeling or delaminated nails. While the nail ideally forms in cohesive layers (see Fig. 1) the cosmetic chemist recruiting consumer panels of typical users has no difficulty finding subjects with severely delaminated nails. This problem is a reality for a large number of nail polish users. Section 5 on multifunctional nail enamel addresses ways to alleviate the problem.

Another problem for the cosmetic chemist to address concerns natural nail moisture. The nail contains from 7 to 12% moisture and passes considerable water every hour [2]. This moisture creates adhesion problems between the nail and decorative nail coatings and can cause the nail to become susceptible to fungal infections if coatings applied are totally occlusive to moisture. Typical nitrocellulose-based nail enamels allow sufficient moisture transfer, which avoids the problem and gives nail enamel an important edge over the typical salon-applied artificial fingernails, which as a rule are impermeable to water vapor.

For a more complete picture of the nail, two technical papers give a more detailed overview [1,2].

2 NAIL STRENGTHENERS

In today's western culture beautiful nails are very much a part of current fashion. Women will go to considerable trouble to develop long nails and, when frustrated, will have artificial nails applied at considerable expense of both time and money. Further, artificial nails for the most part require professional application and maintenance. Yet the demand for beautiful nails is so strong and the ability to grow natural nails so uncertain that nail salons providing application of various artificial nails have become ubiquitous on the American landscape. Most shopping malls have several nail salons specializing in the application and maintenance of these products. Needless to say, the cosmetic chemist and the cosmetics industry have had as a goal the development of a nail treatment that would yield beautiful nails naturally. Formaldehyde treatments have been marketed for this purpose for at least the 35 years that I have been involved in the category [3]. The theory, if there is one, seems to depend upon the ability of formaldehyde to promote polymerization of the keratin by some cross-linking effect. Formaldehyde-containing nail-strengthening products have been available for years. While they may work for some and are legal in most countries despite numerous problems, vast numbers of consumers have resorted to the professional nail salon as the only viable method to get the look of beautiful nails without actually having them. At least with artificial nails you can wear the latest shades of nail enamel and show off beautiful jewelry.

As a cosmetic chemist I have always resisted the pressure to use formaldehyde as a nail strengthener. I have never been able to see tangible results in the panel studies where I have used products containing it as a control. It seems to me that the vague benefits resulting from formaldehyde use fail to justify an ingredient that is a known sensitizer for a great number of people and a possible carcinogen.

An important recent step forward in the nail strengthener category has resulted from a better understanding of how fluoride compounds prevent dental caries when used in toothpaste. Quite simply, fluorides combine with calcium that is part of the tooth structure to form a hard surface, which is then resistant to bacterial attack or acid attack from certain foods. The nail contains calcium as part of its composition, and the chemical attraction between calcium and fluoride is well known.

The cosmetic chemist has failed to recognize the similarity between teeth and nails for years, probably because of the disparity between the calcium concentration in the two materials. Further, the role of calcium as it relates to the texture of the nail has been argued for years. One school of thought attributes the nails' rigid texture to higher calcium levels in the dorsal nail layer, and others feel just as strongly that rigidity must result from the disulfide linkages within the keratin structure [1] Jarrett and Spearman argue for the role of calcium by pointing out that if disulfide linkages were the source of the rigid texture, rodent tails, which contain high levels of disulfide linkages but no calcium, would be rigid [1]. The tooth contains over 30% calcium, whereas the nail contains around 0.1%. While the level of calcium in the nail is low, its role in nail texture is important.

Regardless of any theory, changes in the structure of the nail before and after fluoride treatment are easy to measure by means of a simple but accurate force gauge.

2.1 Measuring Changes in Nail Strength

A simple test developed in our laboratory takes advantage of the semirigidity of the nail, which means that its curvature remains constant for the duration of the test [4]. The finger is placed on a small platform so that the free edge of the nail extends over a mandrel, which has been flattened on the top creating a gap between the top of the mandrel and the nail (Fig. 2.) This distance remains constant during the test period because the curvature of the nail is constant. The force required to flatten the nail against the top of the mandrel is measured with a force gauge. Upon testing the following formula for a fluoride nail treatment from U.S. Patent 5,478,551 [4], it was found that the force required to bend the nail doubled in a 4-week period; data offered in support of the patent were replicated in numerous other tests.

> Formula for a Fluoride Nail Treatment
> Anhydrous ethyl alcohol SDA 40B   98.3%
> Diethylene glycol monomethyl ether   1.0%
> Ammonium hexafluorophosphate   0.7%

In dental products, the monofluorophosphate (MFP) is used. In nail care the hexafluorophosphate offers a number of advantages. Apparently, it is able to form

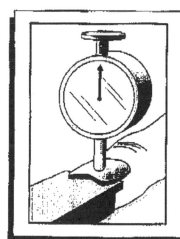

Illustration No. 2
(courtesy J. Buzak, ProStrong, Inc.)

Changes in fingernail strength are easily measured using a simple force gauge. Free edge is extended over flat mandrel and force required to flatten the nail is measured.

FIGURE 2   Changes in fingernail strength are easily measured by using a simple force gauge. The free edge is extended over flat mandrel, and the force required to flatten the nail is measured. (Courtesy of J. Buzak, ProStrong, Inc.)

a better cross-linked network with the low level of calcium in the nail. Ammonium hexafluorophosphate has six fluorine atoms bound to one phosphorus atom forming a diamond-like shape. Since calcium is divalent, it seems possible for one calcium atom to form a bond with two different hexafluorophosphate groups. This is our explanation for the observation that peeling nails grow out in a solid condition after several months of treatment. Further, the hexafluorophosphate is soluble in ethyl alcohol, which makes it convenient to apply: it is very fast drying and does not interfere with the application of nail enamel. As an added benefit, the compound does not release free fluoride ions, making it far less toxic than most fluorides, even many of those commonly used in dentistry. There are several nail treatment products in the current marketplace using this fluoride principle [5]. Further, one of the major cosmetic companies has just announced plans to market a fluoride-based nail treatment within the next year in the mass market. It is therefore likely that this technology will be the treatment of choice as the consumer becomes more aware of its advantages [6].

3 DECORATIVE NAIL COATINGS

This discussion of factors that contribute to multifunctionality refers only tangentially to the manufacture of these products, an area that is left to the specialist equipped to handle the explosive nature of the nitrocellulose primary film formers. Nail coatings by their very nature are multifunctional. While their primary function is purely decorative, they also protect the nail from many environmental elements, including but not limited to water exposure and the many waterborne cleansing materials and chemicals of routine daily life. Nail coatings also give some protection from the physical forces that often go unnoticed until exposure exceeds the physical strength of the nail, resulting in a broken nail. The polish coating can be visualized as a laminate of one or more layers depending on the number of coats and the types of polish used. When enamel is well bonded to the nail, a new structure is created that is stronger than either the uncoated nail or the dry freestanding films. This laminate can be optimized by using several types of polish layered one on top of the other.

This section discusses the three most common coatings making up the laminate structure of a finished manicure: a base coat, a pigmented layer, and a topcoat. While some compromises must be made, it is possible to formulate a single product to function as both base coat and topcoat. Different requirements pertain to each coating, but the three coatings almost always contain common ingredients, and the concentrations are adjusted to obtain the desired function. Table 1 gives examples of ingredients that make up each component of the three types of nail coating. All contain a primary film former (typically nitrocellulose), a modifying

TABLE 1 Ingredients of Typical Nail Coatings

Primary film formers[a]
  Nitrocellulose, 0.25 second RS type
  Nitrocellulose, 0.5 second RS type
  Nitrocellulose, 5–6 second RS type
  Cellulose acetate butyrate, 0.5 second

grades of nitrocellulose are supplied wet with either isopropyl alcohol
or ethyl alcohol. The net amount of dry polymer's 70%; wetting alcohol,
30%.

Secondary film-forming resins
  Sucrose acetate isobutyrate
  Toluenesulfonamide–epoxy resin
  Toluenesulfonamide–formaldehyde resin (used internationally,
  but not in United States)
  Adipic acid–neopental glycol–trimetalic anhydride copolymer

Plasticizers
  Camphor
  Dibutyl phthlate
  Triethyl citrate
  Acetyl triethyl citrate

Active solvents
  Ethyl acetate
  Butyl acetate
  Propyl acetate

Diluents
  Ethyl alcohol, SDA 40B
  Isopropyl alcohol
  n-Heptane

Suspending agents
  Stearalkonium hectocite
  Stearalkonium bentonite

---

[a]Commercial

resin, a plasticizer for the primary film former, and a solvent blend that keeps the
solid ingredients in usable form. For pigmented formula, a suspension blend is
prepared by using a mixture of the foregoing ingredients along with a modified
hectorite or bentonite. The pigments and pearl essence materials used in nail
enamel have been developed over the years and can be found in any of a number
of public domain sources [7].

It can be argued that the base coat is the most important element in a good manicure. The failure of any coating can almost always be attributed primarily to a failure of the base coat.

4 MULTIFUNCTIONALITY IN BASE COATS

The primary function of the base coat is to promote adhesion between the nail and the coatings that follow. Since it is in immediate contact with the nail, the base coat represents an important opportunity to affect the structure of the nail while providing the primary function of adhesion promoter. With some thought, a number of other functions can be provided. These include the following.

1. *Adhesion between layers of delaminated nail.* While the primary function of the base coat is to promote adhesion between the nail and the pigmented enamels that follow, it can also promote adhesion between layers of the nail that have become separated. The dorsal layer of the nail often becomes separated from the intermediate layer, causing both discomfort and an unsightly, unkempt appearance. If this delamination is glued, the nail can grow out in a more sound condition, providing both an important benefit to the user and an important claim for the product. The base coat is the logical product to provide this function. Increasing the polymer solids would be one way to accomplish adhesion between the nail and nail enamel while actually gluing layers of nail together, providing a significant multifunctional base coat.

2. *Maintenance of nail flexibility by balancing nail moisture.* Additional functionality can be developed into the base coat by balancing the permeability of the coating to allow the moisture content of the nail to remain constant. This balance also keeps the nail from becoming too dry and brittle. The moisture passing through the dorsal layer of the nail maintains flexibility that helps prevent broken nails. Most of us have noticed that the nail becomes quite flexible when wet. Trimming nails after bathing is ideal especially for toenails, because the moisture-laden nail is easily trimmed. Conversely, the nail becomes quite brittle when dry. The normal nail passes a considerable amount of moisture, about 1.5 mg of water per square centimeter per hour [8]. If this moisture is not allowed to escape, bonds between the nail and nail enamel are severely weakened. It would be like painting a wet wall with an oil-based paint. When one is formulating a base coat, permeability can be varied by using nitrocellulose as the primary film former and maintaining flexibility by using one of the phthalate esters, which allow good moisture transfer. The modifying resin would be any one of several chosen from Table 1. Permeability is monitored by casting a test film onto a substrate, which allows it to be conveniently lifted when dry. Teflon is a good choice. The freestanding test film is then tested for permeability by means of Method D1653 of the American Society for Testing and Materials (ASTM).

3. *Strengthening the dorsal layer of the nail by forming a matrix between the calcium in the nail and an active ingredient in the base coat.* The dorsal layer of the nail is made up of totally dehydrated cells of hard keratin and contains the highest level of calcium. This calcium can be used to form a reinforcing structure by combining with an active ingredient included there in. See the Busch patents [4,9] for a more complete description of the chemistry between the calcium-containing nail keratin and fluoride compounds. By using a compound such as fluoride to strengthen the nail, the functionality of the base coat is much improved. It will be left to the interested formulator to identify other compounds with similar functionality.

4. *Include ridge-filling ingredients, which help create a smooth beautiful manicure.* Since the surface of the human fingernail becomes rough and uneven, a ridge-filling claim is important for many users of nail enamel. The problem seems to get worse with age. The choice of filler ingredients is broad, but if you choose a heavy ingredient, a suspending agent will be required. Filler ingredients include those commonly used in makeup and include sericite, talc, mica, quartz, and many others [10].

5. *Provide extra cushioning to protect the nail from impact-type forces.* One strategy for formulating a base coat is to increase the polymer solids to improve impact resistance. To this end, more rapidly evaporating solvents are used to reduce the drying time required before additional coats of the manicure are applied.

Summary A base coat formula with multifunctionality can be clearly developed, offering important consumer benefits while providing the marketer with important commercial claims. While the balance of ingredients will be time-consuming to achieve, the benefit to both the consumer and the marketer could well be significant.

5 MULTIFUNCTIONAL PIGMENTED NAIL ENAMEL

As stated earlier, nail enamel is multifunctional by nature. Yet in today's marketplace nail enamel is marketed under two different positionings: therapeutic and fashion. In the fashion positioning any number of niches exist, ranging from plain clear polish to "street colors" favored by kids to elegant frosted enamels worn for special occasions. Most often however, colors are chosen to complement a shade of garment to be worn. This connection between nail enamel colors and fashion trends in clothing requires the marketer of products in this positioning to update shade offerings as often as four times a year. Customers of nail enamel tend to be fashion astute and will buy new shades every season.

In the therapeutically positioned category, an active ingredient is usually included from the group of substances used in the nail-strengthening products discussed later in this chapter. These active ingredients include fluoride compounds, which give strength to the nail by cross-linking with calcium in the nail [9], formaldehyde, which is believed to cross-link with disulfide bonds in the nail, thus increasing nail strength, and higher molecular weight nitrocellulose compounds. You also see advertising for nail polish containing additional gimmicky ingredients that most likely sound more effective than they actually are.

6   MULTIFUNCTIONAL TOPCOATS

The topcoat's primary function is to provide gloss to the manicure [11]. Since it is not usually pigmented, it also offers another layer of strength to the three-layered laminate. The components listed in Table 1 are blended to produce a lacquer with the desired combination of gloss and strength. It is a good idea to consistently use nitrocellulose as the primary film former for all three coating layers, but cellulose acetate butyrate is sometimes used in topcoats because it adheres well to the nitrocellulose layers, has good gloss, and is for the most part nonyellowing [12].

An additional feature can be added to the topcoat by including a small amount of a mirror flake to the clear lacquer [13]. The numerous interesting types available provide a very interesting contrast when used with either an unpigmented base coat or a darker shade of crème nail enamel. The late 1990s saw the introduction of aluminum flakes that appear to be holographic in effect [14]. At any rate, the topcoat can be made more interesting by paying attention to lightweight accent pigments, which add drama and usually require very little or no suspending agent that would compromise the desired gloss level.

7   MULTIFUNCTIONAL NAIL POLISH REMOVER

The primary function of nail polish remover is the utilitarian task of quickly and efficiently removing nail polish. Of course, the formulator must recognize that there are two different types of polish remover in the category. The glue used for acrylic-based artificial nails is adversely affected by acetone, and an "acetone-free" remover is required for these products. The major solvent in the acetone-free category is ethyl acetate, which can be used for either natural nails or acrylics. At any rate, the method for screening moisturizing or conditioning agents is the same for either type of remover. For natural nails, acetone is the solvent of choice, and it is quite capable of extracting water and some of the natural oils from the nails and cuticle, leaving the nail brittle and the cuticle around the nail dry and irritated. It is my belief that many broken nails are caused by the damaging effects of polish remover.

While polish remover is not intentionally applied to the cuticle, contact is almost unavoidable, and dry irritated cuticles result. Since our company sells fingernail treatments, we are particularly interested in avoiding damage to the newly strengthened nail. Many of our customers have nails of normal length for the first time and are more than willing to pay a premium for a polish remover that not only avoids damage but actually treats the nail and cuticle with ingredients that keep the nail flexible and cuticle well conditioned. Polish remover that has been formulated with both functions assigned a high priority may cost more than the traditionally low-priced products in the category, but it need not be expensive compared with a typical hand lotion or cream. After a customer has gone to the time and expense of developing beautiful nails, protecting those nails from damage is a major concern for both our customer and our company. We assign a very high priority to both functions, and our polish remover has enjoyed considerable success even though it costs more than many products in the marketplace. That said, product lines wishing to maintain a high-quality image must perform their primary remover function extremely well.

Polish remover becomes multifunctional when it performs its primary function quickly and contains conditioners that improve the texture of the fingernail, moisturize and condition the cuticle area around the nail, or both. Nail polish remover is one of the simpler of the nail care products to formulate, so there is not much excuse for a bad formula. Even so, the products recently reviewed in today's marketplace either removed polish or conditioned the nail and cuticle but not both. To accomplish the primary function of polish removal, solvents are used that are by their very nature damaging to the nail and the tissue surrounding the nail. Therefore, the formulator has several choices. One is to use enough solvent to efficiently remove polish and not worry about the consequences. A second is to dilute the solvent, minimizing the damage but providing a barely functional product. A third is a combination of both, that is, an attempt to provide functionality and some conditioning in the same product.

Most products in the current marketplace claim the latter: they claim to use ingredients that are beneficial, which is accurate; but most have also diluted activity, causing a major decrease in polish removal time. For acetone-based products, the primary conditioning agent in the majority of products seems to be water. There is some logic for including water as an ingredient, and we use it as well; the use level in typical products recently purchased, however, dramatically reduced the removal efficiency. It makes one wonder whether the main consideration was cost rather than replacing or minimizing the negative effects of acetone. While the traditional retail price of polish remover is low, it is possible both to provide excellent functionality and to meet relatively stringent cost considerations.

Multifunctional polish removers using either acetone or ethyl acetate as the active solvent include ingredients that overcome the drying effects of the solvents and treat the cuticle, which has become dry and irritated. While every ingredient added to a formula other than the active solvent increases the time and effort required to remove polish, small amounts can be included to mitigate the drying effects of the chosen solvent. Since water is totally miscible with acetone, amounts of up to 10% are usually included in removers of these types to provide hydration and retard undue water depletion due to the acetone. Even at levels up to 10%, the removal effectiveness is not overly reduced and the hydration benefit is real. Ethyl acetate is able to absorb up to 3% water, and small amounts are included in this type of formula to provide some hydration of the nail. Since ethyl acetate does not directly extract water from the nail, a 3% inclusion is a meaningful amount.

A wide range of moisturizing ingredients that provide conditioning and moisturization of the nail and cuticle can be included. Ingredients used to moisturize and condition the nail and cuticle are chosen based on their solubility in the active solvent. Almost any therapeutic ingredient useful in other skin care products can be used in nail polish remover. While it is customary to use moisturizers and conditioners that are inexpensive because nail polish remover is typically one of the lowest priced items in the beauty department, it is prudent to use one that provides the maximum effectiveness at the lowest concentration. This strategy provides maximum treatment with the least negative impact on product performance. The test method that follows allows one to create a balance between removal efficiency, cost, and treatment of nail and cuticle.

The formulation strategy for polish remover is to choose a target remover efficiency end point and then screen ingredients to identify those that provide maximum benefit at the lowest cost. While it has been customary to use consumer panel evaluations to evaluate polish remover in vivo, the following in vitro method has proved to be quite reliable, and its results correlate well with results from consumer panels. When human panels are used, it is important that panelists wear the nail polish for at least 24 hours before removal. A major advantage of the in vitro method is that the test substrate is fully cured and tests can be performed at any time. By performing the in vitro test, we can screen any number of moisturizing and conditioning ingredients, making sure that remover efficiency is not compromised.

8   METHOD FOR TESTING NAIL POLISH REMOVER EFFICIENCY

8.1   Background

Since the primary film former used to formulate nail enamel is nitrocellulose, a nitrocellulose membrane filter is used as the test substrate. These membrane filters have been developed for use in certain microbiological assays and are readily available from any scientific catalog. They have a very well controlled pore size, and when a constant volume of test product is dropped on their surface, the time required to dissolve the filter is very reproducible. When either acetone or ethyl acetate serves as the active remover ingredient, the undiluted solvent can be used as a control.

8.2 Equipment

The removal efficiency test calls for the following equipment.

Stopwatch
Microliter syringe (10 μL)
Membrane filter nitrocellulose, Schleicher & Schuell, 0.45 μm or equivalent

8.3 Test Method

Using the undiluted active solvent as a control, fill the syringe with 2 μL of solvent. Position membrane filter on a flat surface and discharge 2 μL of liquid from the syringe. The small drop of liquid will accumulate on the tip of the syringe needle. Transfer the measured drop of liquid to the membrane surface while starting the stopwatch. A clear circle will develop in the nitrocellulose membrane, which is normally opaque. Repeat the test for a total of three measurements. Record the time required to reach the clear-circle end point. The average of the three measurements gives the time required for the trial formula to dissolve the test nitrocellulose sample. While we still perform typical panel evaluations on formulas that are close to being marketed, I have never seen a formula that tested satisfactorily on this test fail with consumers. When comparing results of a test formula with the undiluted solvent, the end-point times of the sample may even double that of the solvent before the consumer will object. Of course it is important to choose a control that the consumer accepts and make judgments about the proposed formula based on this type of comparison.

Test volumes and the pore size of the filter can be varied depending on availability as long as the standard and sample are run in the same way. In the test just described, acetone will produce the end point in 11 seconds. Ethyl acetate produces the same end point in 7 seconds. A well-formulated nail polish remover using acetone as the active solvent will produce the end point in 18–19 seconds. In my opinion the ingredients used to dilute the active solvent and provide additional multifunctional benefits should not exceed an end point 21 seconds. In 2001 I tested most of the mass-marketed removers and found that about half exceeded that point, with several requiring more that a minute to dissolve the membrane. Removers with an end point of 20.2 seconds were determined to be highly effective when tested in the traditional in vivo panel mode.

Nonacetone products are used to remove polish from artificial nails because acetone can damage the adhesive used with these products. The solvent of choice for this type of product is ethyl acetate. Ethyl acetate, while less dehydrating than acetone, can still extract lipids from the cuticle area, causing the skin to actually show white striations where the natural oils have been extracted. Further, ethyl acetate creates a regulatory issue because it is considered to be a volatile organic compound (VOC) by both the U.S. Environmental Protection Agency and the state of California. Both have limits on its use. At the time of writing, the limit was 75%, but the regulations change quite often, and it is always prudent to monitor both the federal requirements [15] and California Air Resources web site [16].

Choose a primary solvent based on whether the product is for natural nails or artificial nails. Then choose a moisturizer and conditioning group of ingredients based on desired marketing claims, solubility of ingredient in the primary solvent, cost-effectiveness, and performance at the lowest concentration. Popular ingredients include aloe, glycerin, lanolin and its derivatives, the myristates, vitamin E acetate, panthenol, and arachdyl propionate. Of course new moisturizers are introduced every day and can be good choices when supported by the manufacturer's efficacy data as well as meeting the other criteria for use.

9   MULTIFUNCTIONAL CUTICLE TREATMENTS

The primary function of cuticle treatment products has changed somewhat over the years. Thirty years ago the emphasis was limited to cuticle removers that aided in pushing back or even dissolving the part of the cuticle, which extends over the base of the nail. Ingredients used for this purpose were very harsh and included potassium hydroxide at a high level. While these products still exist, the primary function and emphasis have become broader and more practical. Cuticle products are now positioned to treat most of the skin tissue that immediately comes in contact with the fingernail. Our own line of nail care products includes several cuticle treatments, none of which contain potassium hydroxide. This change of emphasis offers the consumer products that are more helpful in dealing with real conditions, including hangnails, broken irritated skin where hangnails have been removed, and the thick accumulations of dry skin that form around the sides of the nail.

Multifunctionality can be achieved by including ingredients that can help with the original problem of removing skin tissue from the nail surface and also help with problem skin on the sides of the fingernail. One choice would be the inclusion of an α-hydroxy acid buffered to a fairly low pH value (pH 4 is effective for a daily use product). When combined with traditional moisturizing ingredients, multifunctionality is obtained where really needed.

α-Hydroxy acids have been very popular in facial treatment products, where they aid in removing layers of dead skin cells, creating a softer, younger looking skin. The α-hydroxy phenomenon in facial treatment has become a standard in the category because the effect is real in a category where the benefit beyond moisturization has seldom been readily apparent even in products tagged with a high retail price. This exfoliation process is extremely useful on the cuticle, where thick cracked skin surrounding the nail is an unfortunate reality for many consumers. Further, when this exfoliation process is used on a regular basis, it accomplishes the objectives of the original potassium hydroxide products with a much milder formula. When α-hydroxy acid products are used daily for a week or so, the skin is removed from the surface of the nail in small amounts rather than as a single step, but the harshness of the potassium hydroxide product is avoided. A major benefit is the gradual removal of the heavy thick skin on the sides of the nail, where hangnails and the like become a problem. While users should be advised not to use any cosmetic product on broken, bleeding skin, daily use of α-hydroxy treatments will not cause such breaches in the integrity of the skin.

Another approach to multifunctionality in the cuticle category would be the use of ingredients that can truly protect the skin from the harsh ingredients of daily life. Washing the hands a number of times per day, not to mention routine use of typical household cleaners, puts quite a strain on the skin of the hands. In the United States, the use of 1–10% dimethicone qualifies the product as a skin protectant, as does the use of petrolatum and several other ingredients. If skin protectant claims are made, the product might be considered an over-the-counter drug and will be required to conform with the monograph for such products published in the *Federal Register* [15]. Such a product is very helpful, however, when the skin in this area becomes truly irritated.

Suggested α-hydroxy acid ingredients include glycolic acid and lactic acid at levels from 4 to 7%, neutralized with either triethanolamine or aminomethyl propanol.

Ingredients qualifying as skin protectants for this type of product are dimethicone (1–30%), glycerin (20–45%), petrolatum (30–100%), shark liver oil (0.3%), and white petrolatum (30–100%).

REFERENCES

1. A Jarrett, RIC Spearman. The histochemistry of the human nail. Arch Dermatol 94 (November 1966).
2. GV Gupchup, JL Zatz. Structural characteristics and permeability of the human nail: A review. J Cosmet Sci. 50(6): 363–385 (1999).
3. JB Wilkinson, RJ Moore. Harry's Cosmeticology. New York: Chemical Publishing, 1982, p 372.
4. FW Busch Jr. Non-aqueous composition for hardening and strengthening fingernails and toenails. US Patent 5,478,551 (1995).
5. JB Devos. Method of hardening and strengthening keratin and composition. US Patent 4,919,920 (1990).
6. F-D-C Reports. Rose Sheet, 21(27): 4 (July 2000).
7. P Delmonica. EPA and state regulation of volatile organic compounds. In: NF Estrin and JM Akerson, eds. Cosmetic Regulation in a Competitive Environment. New York: Marcel Dekker, 2000, pp 91–93.

8. D Spruit. Measurement of water loss through human nail in vivo, J Invest Dermatol. 56: 359–361 (1971).
9. FW Busch, KA Therrien. Long wearing fingernail enamels containing fluoride compounds. US Patent 5,811,084 (1998).
10. M Kobayashi M Taizo. Sericite: A functional filler. Cosmet Toiletries 115(8) (August 2000).
11. WP Smith. Hydroxy acids and skin aging. Cosmet Toiletries 109 (September 1994).
12. Cellulose Acetate Butyrate. In: World of Eastman Chemicals, Technical Bulletin P-160H. Rochester, NY: Eastman, 1995.
13. AA Patil, RW Sandewicz. Nail lacquer technology. In: Monograph No. 6, Society of Cosmetic Chemist. New York: SCC, 2000, pp 21–23.
14. Spectratek Technologies, Inc. Technical bulletin (1994). www.spectratek.net, http://www.spectratek.net.
15. Fed Regist 63(176) (Sept 11, 1998).

7

Cosmeceuticals: Combining Cosmetic and Pharmaceutical Functionality

Billie L. Radd
BLR Consulting Services, Naperville, Illinois, U.S.A.

1 INTRODUCTION

All cosmeceutical products are multifunctional. The term "cosmeceutical" conveys that a product has characteristics combining the aesthetic appeal and benefits of traditional cosmetic products with a therapeutic component. The therapeutic component can be associated, in the strictest sense, with pharmaceutical products. It is a much needed term to describe cosmetic products that have some therapeutic advantage over traditional cosmetics, yet are not drug products.

Although the use of the term "cosmeceutical" seems like a simplistic designation to describe the products that bridge the characteristics of cosmetics to drug products (Fig. 1), there is a multifaceted controversy over the use of the term. Key points that contribute to issues surrounding the use of the term "cosmeceutical" include the following.

1. The U.S. Food and Drug Administration (FDA) has established separate definitions for cosmetics and pharmaceuticals. These definitions govern U.S. laws. The FDA does not acknowledge the term "cosmeceutical" [1].

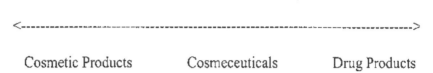

Cosmetic Products   Cosmeceuticals   Drug Products

Figure 1 A continuum between cosmetics and pharmaceutical products. (From Ref. 1.)

2. The European Union has established different European Court (EC) directives that separately discuss cosmetics and drugs [2]. There is no provision for the term "cosmeceutical." Most of the national regulations for cosmetics and drugs agree with the definitions set forth in the EC directives.
3. The term "cosmeceutical" was introduced in 1961 by Raymond E. Reed and popularized in years to follow by Albert M. Kligman, MD, Ph.D. [1,3]. As of the year 2001, no official consensus for a definition of cosmeceutical existed within the cosmetic, toiletry, or pharmaceutical industry, nor was one close to being established [1,2,4,5].

"Cosmeceutical" has been used to describe products that yield benefits traditionally thought to be cosmetic in nature, such as moisturization, as well as products that make marketing claims approaching those of drug products, such as reducing (the appearance of) wrinkles. It has been suggested that the term be used to classify cosmetics of different types [2]. Japan was progressive in attempting to make such a new product classification, referred to as "quasi-drugs" [1,2]. The new classification included substances causing "a mild action on the body" and demonstrated to be safe. There remains much controversy over how to classify and register products into this new classification, without a major advantage for doing so.

2   A HISTORICAL SUMMARY OF DRUG AND COSMETIC TERMS

The Food, Drug and Cosmetic (FDC) Act of 1938 was enacted after more than 40 persons died upon ingesting the drug sulfanilamide in a toxic formulation containing diethylene glycol [6,7]. The FDC Act set forth requirements for the testing of products and their components to ensure they are safe for human use. It also clearly defined the terms.

Drug: A substance intended to be used in the cure, diagnosis, mitigation, prevention, or treatment of disease in man or in other animals. It is a non-food substance that affects the structure or function of the human body or of animals [1,6,7].

Cosmetic: A substance applied to the human body for the purpose of altering the appearance, beautifying, cleansing, or promoting attractiveness.
Soaps do not fall under the definition of cosmetics [1,6].

Note that if a product is classified as both a cosmetic and a drug, it must meet the
regulatory requirements for both cosmetics and drugs [1].

The FDA was created in 1938 to administer and enforce the FDC Act. In
1962, after the drug thalidomide was found to cause birth defects, the FDC Act
was amended to require a greater amount of safety testing for drug products, as
well as proof that drugs are effective to treat indicated ailments [7]. From a regulatory standpoint, courts follow the definitions and requirements outlined in the
FDC Act in then evaluations of drug and cosmetic products, including product
components, claims, labeling, and advertising [1]. The EC directives serve a similar purpose in Europe.

3 REGULATIONS VERSUS TIME AND TECHNOLOGY

Recalling that the FDC Act was written in 1938, it becomes obvious that major
technological findings have substantially increased our knowledge about human
physiology, as well as product formulation and function [1,2,4,5]. Now clinical
techniques are available that will demonstrate how substances such as water and
petrolatum, once thought to be inactive, alter the structure and function of skin [5].
For practical reasons, the FDA does not require such substances to be reclassified
as drugs. Instead, it typically determines when cosmetic products need to be
reclassified based on manufacturers' claims about the products.

3.1 Pharmaceutical Classification

As just summarized, all drugs must submit proven safety and efficacy data before
receiving FDA marketing approval. A very time-consuming and expensive
process has evolved for demonstrating the safety and efficacy of a new drug [7]. A
"Notice of Claimed Investigational Exemption for a New Drug" (IND) must be
filed and approved by the FDA before the substance can be clinically tested on
humans. At this time, a multiphase protocol for drug testing must be submitted and
approved. If testing proves appropriate, the manufacturer can file a New Drug
Application (NDA). The NDA presents all the testing data gathered on the drug.
The process takes an average of 12 years, and has escalating estimates for
expenses. When NDA approval has been granted, the new drug can be marketed.
Note that the manufacturer is required to continue to gather clinical information
about the drug after marketing it, and to report these data to the FDA. If the manufacturer wishes to modify the delivery system of the drug, an Abbreviated New
Drug Application (ANDA) must be filed and approved.

When an NDA is approved, the FDA determines if the drug should be available via a physician's prescription or made available to the public "over the counter" (OTC: i.e., without a prescription) [6]. If a drug is habit forming, is not safe for self-medication, is potentially hazardous, is new and has not completed its safety testing, or presents uncertainties in its administration, it will be classified as a prescription drug. Medications that do not fall under these restrictions are made available to the public as OTC medications. Many OTC drugs were introduced as prescription medications, then reclassified after confirming results of safety testing and consumer use information had been reviewed. Note that the introduction of new OTC medications into the marketplace requires the manufacturer to complete the IND/NDA approval process.

3.2 Cosmetic Classification

Cosmetic products are not required to undergo the extensive testing described for drug products, and the regulations governing their labeling, manufacturing, and distribution are much more relaxed [8]. The FDA cannot require cosmetic manufacturers to disclose information about their manufacturing plants, register their products, document information about the ingredients used in their products, track and report adverse reactions to their products, or test their products for safety and efficacy. The FDA, however, keeps track of adverse reaction information it receives from consumers, hospitals, physician surveys, and manufacturers that voluntarily report such data. It keeps a database that is searchable by product brand name, manufacturer, product type, associated injuries, and formulation number (when the manufacturer voluntarily registers a formula).

Upon noting the differences in regulatory requirements between drug and cosmetic products, it becomes obvious that it is substantially less time-consuming and costly to introduce a new cosmetic into the marketplace than a prescription or OTC drug. To maintain some consistency within the cosmetic and toiletry industry, the Cosmetic, Toiletry, and Fragrance Association (CTFA) was created to work with and on behalf of the cosmetic manufacturers. Some of its functions include acting as a liaison between manufacturers and the FDA, helping to propose and secure the adoption of industry standards, proposing simplified cosmetic ingredient labeling names, reviewing ingredient safety and toxicity data, and aiding manufacturers in meeting FDA label requirements.

3.3 Product Classification

The FDA essentially determines whether a cosmetic product should be reclassified as a drug based on the claims that are made about the product [1]. Without ever formally acknowledging that portions of the FDC Act are obsolete, the FDA is nevertheless fairly flexible when reviewing cosmetic claims. To date, it more often has chosen to issue warning letters rather than recalls to manufacturers when claims become too druglike. As a result, many cosmetic products make therapeutic claims to varying degrees, without the manufacturers taking the required time and expense to prove product safety and efficacy.

3.4 Views Regarding the Term "Cosmeceutical"

An aspect of the cosmeceutical revolution to consider is its reason for being in the first place. Historically, consumer needs and demands have driven the cosmetic market to evolve to this point. Many years ago, a cosmetic or toiletry product was expected to have one simple function. For example, a lotion helped to moisturize dry skin, and a deodorant was used to mask body odors. As consumers increasingly demanded substantially more benefits from cosmetics and toiletries, multifunctional products were born [1,2]. For example, now a moisturizing lotion also may have antiitch benefits, promote skin exfoliation to reduce flakiness, and promote the healing of dry skin by supplying substances essential to maintain the barrier layer function. Most deodorants now are also OTC drugs because they contain antiperspirants to keep underarms dry in addition to masking body odors.

Intense competition between companies, coupled with expressed consumer social needs, tempt manufacturers to push cosmeceutical product claims as close as possible to the drug definition, without adopting it [1,2]. To illustrate the transition from cosmetic product claims to multifunctional cosmeceutical claims, Table 1 lists some terms that convey benefits historically considered to be purely cosmetic, as well as terms that might be considered to be more cosmeceutical in nature [8].

Many industry professionals agree that there is a need for a term to describe products that moved beyond the simplistic cosmetic definition but for practical purposes are not drugs [2,4,5]. For some, the term "cosmeceutical" meets that

TABLE 1 Cosmetic Versus Cosmeceutical Terms That Convey Product Benefits

Cosmetic terms	Cosmeceutical term
Moisturizes, rehydrates, protects	Prevents signs of aging, antiaging
Beautifies, conceals, highlights, enhances	Reduces the appearance of fine lines and wrinkles
Softens, conditions, lubricates	Regenerates damaged skin
Smoothes rough skin	Firms
Absorbs excess skin oils	Heals, stimulates skin repair
Cleanses, tones, refreshes, clarifies	Penetrates into the skin to act
Deodorizes	Fades hyperpigmentation spots

Source: Ref. 8.

need. Cosmetic and toiletry industry professionals agree that they do not want to create circumstances under which their products will become reclassified as drugs. At present, cosmetic products are quickly and cost-effectively introduced to market. The reclassification of cosmetic products to drugs would require that they become subject to the expensive and time-consuming drug approval process. This would seriously jeopardize the future of the cosmetic and toiletry industry. Within the industry, however, there is little consensus regarding the extent of allowable cosmetic efficacy claims. It is the implications of product efficacy and the extent of associated claims that create the heart of the cosmeceutical controversy [2].

The more risks associated with using a product, the greater the justification for regulating the product more closely. If a manufacturer wants to consider an efficacy claim for a cosmetic product, the extent of the claim should be examined [2]. If the claim implies a local effect, FDA action will probably be less likely than it would with respect to a claim that implies a systemic effect. For example, if a topical product claims to penetrate deep into skin tissues to cause a biological response, it is reasonable to assume that a systemic effect can result from the product usage. Greater systemic effects imply greater safety risks to consumers using the products. Consumer safety is one of the ultimate concerns of the FDA. Owing to the nature of their use, the safety testing requirements for cosmetic products are minimal [2]. Industry standards, however, advocate that cosmetic products contain ingredients that have adequate safety testing. To preserve the regulatory status that cosmetics and toiletries now enjoy, manufacturers wanting to make assertive efficacy claims for cosmetic products must be responsible to conduct product safety testing beyond the minimum.

In summary, the term "cosmeceutical" will most likely continue to be used for years to come [1,2,5]. It indicates that a particular product is multifunctional because it combines both cosmetic and drug functionalities. A popular example of such a product is a facial moisturizer that is an OTC sunscreen that helps prevent photoaging. Because international opinions and regulations are ever changing, the probability that "cosmeceutical" will be adopted as an official regulatory term is questionable. One thing that is certain, however: as the technology evolution continues, cosmetic products also will evolve, and the issues just discussed will remain lively topics of debate.

4 DEVELOPING COSMECEUTICAL PRODUCTS

As stated in the opening paragraph of this chapter, all cosmeceuticals are multifunctional because they have both cosmetic and therapeutic properties. Since consumers demand that more than one need be met by each cosmeceutical product, the very multifunctionality of cosmeceutical creates a wide range of variation among these products. The focus of this discussion will be to outline considerations for developing cosmeceutical products that have various multifunctional benefits. Ingredient categories that are recognized as being used in cosmeceutical products to yield some of the multifunctional benefits also are highlighted. The details involved with combining specific ingredients are discussed thoroughly in the references provided at the end of this chapter. By following the recommendations presented in this chapter, and consulting the references as needed, a formulator should be able to efficiently evaluate the feasibility of using active ingredients in combination with each other to create a multifunctional cosmeceutical product.

4.1 Defining the Desired Product

Before any product can be made, the formulator must know what criteria are essential for the desired product's success [9]. This helps keep development efforts focused and leads to more efficient product introductions. Ideally, the formulator should get information on the following categories.

Product concept: A product is best designed if the following items are clearly understood: the needs and expectations of consumers who will be using the product, the products that will compete with the new product in the marketplace, and whether the new product needs to fit within a line of products.

Product type: Knowing the physical form of the product is essential to developing any formulation plan. Different product forms require different ingredients, and they have different stability requirements and processing needs. In addition, the therapeutic benefits achieved from product usage will change with type of form chosen [7]. Product parameters such as fragrance needs, type of package, special use conditions, and unique claims desired also should be discussed.

Required ingredients: Since cosmeceuticals are multifunctional, there often are a variety of ingredients that must be included in the product to maximize the therapeutic value and associated claims for the product. Any ingredients necessary to support the product concept or intended marketing claims must be identified before the start of formulation. Note that to yield therapeutic benefits, many ingredients must be used at specified quantities and require special formulation techniques. For this reason, it is critical that formulations be designed around the required ingredients to maximize their stability and efficacy.

Ingredients to omit: Ingredients that may interfere with the therapeutic functions of the required ingredients must be omitted. Ingredients that do not fit with the product concept also must not be considered for the new formulation. For example, a fragrance cannot be put into a product marketed as fragrance free, and ingredients that might contribute to a bad odor in an unfragranced base must be omitted.

Product performance: Cosmeceutical products must deliver a therapeutic benefit as well as meeting the aesthetic expectations of the consumer. These multifunctional requirements typically necessitate a battery of tests to measure the product performance in both respects. In general, purely pharmaceutical products may succeed with being therapeutic only. The multifunctional demands on cosmeceuticals, however, require that they yield therapeutic benefits while being pleasing to use. This goal is technically challenging for many product types. For example, it took years to develop aesthetic antiperspirant products that did not turn white after application onto the skin. Superior multifunctional product performance is so important that most manufacturers commonly measure product prototype performance attributes versus identified competitive products throughout the development process.

Regulatory input: The regulatory organization should outline policies that may affect the product formulation and testing, such as active levels, stability needs, marketing claims, and issues to consider for international marketing.

Timetable: A project team that has representatives from key parts of the organization should develop a joint plan that outlines important dates and costs associated with moving the product into the marketplace. Expressed developmental needs should at least include formulation time, processing and scale-up time, stability needs, and time to conduct clinical and sensory testing. Initial agreement on a plan typically results in an efficient project execution and is beneficial in reducing rework.

4.2 Formulating with Active Ingredients

Since cosmeceutical products are multifunctional, they typically contain more than one active ingredient. The combination of actives contributes to the multiple claimed benefits associated with product usage. Cosmeceutical actives can be considered to be ingredients whose functions are to provide benefits to the consumer. The choice of ingredients that may be used as actives in cosmeceutical products is extensive enough to preclude a complete listing in this chapter. Instead, the general concepts important to consider when formulating with most actives are discussed, along with special ingredient categories that contain commonly used therapeutic actives. The benefits that result from using a product containing the specified actives often include, but are not limited to, a combination of the ones listed in Table 1. Note that it is not uncommon to find OTC drug and cosmeceutical product combinations, such as facial creams that contain sunscreens. These products are both drugs and cosmetics, hence must meet all the regulatory demands for both categories.

Formulating multifunctional products requires a planned, organized approach to building a product. If a rational process is embraced, active incompatibilities and instabilities are more easily recognized, permitting technical challenges to be addressed promptly and logically. The first step in cosmeceutical formulation is identifying the most appropriate actives to include in the product [9]. Once identified, the following parameters must be evaluated.

4.2.1   Physical and Chemical Properties of Active Ingredients

To yield a therapeutic benefit, an active ingredient must remain stable from the time of product production until the consumer finishes the product. The physical and chemical properties of the active dictate the necessity for special conditions or formulation techniques to maintain stability [3,9]. Key properties to consider include molecular size, pH, ionization parameters, buffer capacity or requirements, partition coefficient, volatility, melting point, solubility, odor, and color. Often this information is available from ingredient suppliers or in published texts [6,7,10,11]. Heat, light, and moisture stability should be evaluated if published information is not available. Differences in active properties between production lots or manufacturers should be noted.

When combining actives to create multifunctional cosmeceutical products, a logical first step is to evaluate these parameters for each active to determine whether there are any conflicts between the properties of different active ingredients. If a conflict is found, then the formulator must determine whether there are ways to meet the needs for the actives within one product or whether the conflict is so profound that the actives cannot be used together. For example, if one active requires a low pH to remain stable and deliver a therapeutic benefit from the product, and a second active requires a high product pH, the two actives may not be able to be used in the same product. However, if one active deactivates another active, there may be a way of encapsulating or protecting one of the actives in such a way that both will remain stable in the product.

4.2.2   Safety of Active Ingredients

The irritation potential of an active to skin and eyes, along with toxicity information, should be documented. If irritation or toxicity problems are suspected, the ability to correct these issues within the formulation must be assessed. Issues with delivering an appealing product based on safety information about its actives should be promptly brought to the attention of the project team.

Since multiple actives often are used in cosmeceuticals, the irritation potential and toxicity profiles of the individual actives may be influenced by the other actives in the combination. In addition, some active irritation potentials and toxicity profiles may shift relative to the other ingredients and formulation properties. For example, some α-hydroxy acid ingredients are substantially more irritating at lower pH values. As a result, it is prudent to screen the safety and toxicity of the product prototype formulations to identify the best pH to meet the therapeutic requirements for the product without jeopardizing the safety of the user.

4.2.3   Concentration of Active Ingredients

Before discussing concentration, it is necessary to note that the absorption of actives after topical application depends on many factors other than the product formulation [1,7,9,12]. These include the site of application and region of the body, the size of the application site, the degree of skin hydration, the condition of the skin, the amount of time the product is in contact with the application site, how the product is applied to the site, the frequency of product application, and the use of occlusive dressings over the site of application. Active absorption into the skin is a subject of much debate [13]. Cosmeceuticals should penetrate into the skin, but not through the skin. If an active penetrates through the skin to enter the systemic circulation and cause body-wide effects, it may be classified as a drug. Some formulation considerations for active concentration are outlined next.

Concentration of the Active Ingredient at the Delivery Site. Since cosmeceuticals often contain more than one active ingredient, one must consider the possible alternatives that dictate the concentration of each active. Under ideal conditions, the actives will not interact with each other, or with other ingredients in the product. This allows each active to be considered as an independent source yielding a therapeutic benefit.

If the actives interact in some way, rather than acting independently, a number of assessments must be made. If they act synergistically to produce the therapeutic effect, it may be possible to reduce the essential concentration of the actives needed at the delivery site. If they act synergistically to produce an unwanted effect, such as irritation, their concentration may need to be reduced to ensure that consumers will be able to tolerate product usage.

If the actives behave antagonistically, it may be possible to incorporate them into the product at a higher essential concentration to yield therapeutic benefits. Often, however, the actives react and become inactivated. In such cases, specialized active delivery systems, such as encapsulation systems, may help keep the actives stable in the formulation. Note that the challenge of working with these systems lies in assuring that the actives are released at the site of delivery during application in order to produce their effect.

Sometimes marketers may want to include more than one active from the same ingredient class in a product. Even though the actives are coming from the same class, they must be evaluated individually, then collectively, to determine how they will affect the therapeutic value of the product. For example, most α-hydroxy acid actives deliver similar therapeutic effects with varying amounts of associated irritation. The extent of the final product therapeutic effect must be evaluated to ensure that the combination of acid actives delivers the therapeutic benefits without making the product too irritating. Different vitamins, however, not only deliver very different therapeutic effects, but have very different physical property and formulation requirements, as well. While the individual therapeutic effects for each vitamin must be verified, the formulation focus should be to ensure that each vitamin active is compatible and stable in the product.

Some active ingredients are inherently multifunctional and can render more than one therapeutic benefit. Sometimes the type of benefit realized is a function of the concentration of the active. For example, urea is known as a moisturizer. At higher concentrations it relieves itching, and at the highest concentrations it is very irritating and used to treat wounds. Antioxidants comprise another example: used therapeutically in cosmeceutical products to help prevent free radicals from damaging skin cells, they also help preserve the product.

There are a variety of other ingredients that may be added to formulations that can enhance the therapeutic effect of actives at the delivery site. Examples of such ingredients include penetration enhancers, film formers, and solubilizers. Ingredients such as anti-irritants may work to diminish unwanted active attributes without adversely impacting the therapeutic benefits of the actives. The need for ingredients of these types varies with the cost and performance expectations of the actives. If such ingredients are needed, their impact on the performance of the entire product should be evaluated. If ingredients that detract from the performance of the product actives are added to the formulation, they should be eliminated if possible. If better ingredient substitutions cannot be made, then specialized delivery systems for the actives should be considered. The impact of such ingredients on the performance of the entire product should be evaluated.

Finally, the type of product form and use conditions typically dictate how much active gets delivered to the site of action from the product, and how much time the active has to achieve its effect. Thus, a change in product form or use conditions may dictate a change in the product active concentration.

Active Ingredient Concentration Needed in the Product. The active concentration in the product must be maintained until the consumer has finished the product. Again, since cosmeceuticals are multifunctional and often contain more than one active, the stability of each active in the product must be carefully evaluated to ensure that the minimum amount of each active needed to produce a therapeutic response is present throughout the product use period.

4.2.4 Active Forms

Actives often are available in different forms. For example, actives that are acids or bases may be available as salts, and some actives are available in polar or non-polar vehicles. Note that different active forms often have different abilities to produce the desired therapeutic effect, as well as different stabilities. For example, the vitamin A esters are more physically stable than vitamin A, but the therapeutic benefits of vitamin A versus those from vitamin A esters vary. Once the ability of a form to produce an effect has been demonstrated, the required active concentration in the product can be determined. If active forms are interchanged, the resultant changes in active concentration must be determined.

In summary, when multiple actives are incorporated into a product, the actives must either be compatible or be delivered in such a way that they will remain stable enough to impart therapeutic benefits for the life of the product. Evaluating which active forms meet both therapeutic and formulation stability requirements prior to developing the final product is the most efficient approach to formulating multifunctional products.

4.2.5   Special Ingredient Categories Used in Multifunctional Cosmeceuticals

There are many actives currently used in multifunctional cosmeceutical products, and new ones are being promoted as fast as the industry can reasonably consider their use. A casual review of the ingredient lists and claims of marketed multifunctional cosmeceutical products makes it obvious that the trend is to push formulators to include in a product as many actives as possible to attempt to meet a particular consumer need. The challenge of multifunctional product formulation is to evaluate the feasibility of combining these actives, and to create products that yield the expected therapeutic benefits. This, as outlined earlier, depends on the specific physical attributes of the actives and the required product aesthetic parameters. If the actives can be delivered in unison and will meet the product performance requirements, only the imagination can limit what types of multifunctionality will result from active combinations. Thus it is not practical to discuss the possible combinations of active ingredients. The active combinations often are dictated by product niche, consumer receptiveness, and marketing creativity.

The limitations for multiple active use typically are associated with either safety or incompatibility issues. For example, it is well known that α-hydroxy acid products can be very irritating to the delicate tissues associated with the lips, eyes, and mucous membranes. Depending upon the pH of and active concentration in such products, severe damage may occur with inappropriate use. As a result, the development of a α-hydroxy acid product that would be positioned for use around the eyes or lips seems remote, unless an effective nonirritating formulation can be developed with substantial safety data to promote its use.

There have been numerous product suggestions that seem logical to the nontechnical community but are not technically feasible. Technical product limitations must be acknowledged, although they are not fondly embraced by nontechnical personnel. For example, creating an aqueous spray solution that contains an active that is unstable in water is not technically feasible. Alternatives to this concept can be explored with the idea source, but executing this exact idea as presented is not possible. As techniques for active delivery systems are enhanced, and unique package delivery systems are developed, the marketing of such products may one day become a reality.

Following are examples of some special ingredient categories that contain therapeutic actives that commonly have been used in multifunctional cosmeceutical products. The details for formulating these actives in combination with each other to create multifunctional products are beyond the scope of this chapter. By referring to the formulation principles already outlined, and then consulting the references cited at the end of this chapter, a reasonable assessment can be made for combining specific actives into desired products.

Antioxidants. Antioxidants (AOs) prevent harmful oxygen species, also called free radicals, from damaging skin cells and accelerating aging. Cosmeceutical products sometimes incorporate AO ingredients to enhance product stability. It is not uncommon to find more than one AO in a cosmeceutical formulation, with some of the actives being included for therapeutic value and others for product stability. For example, many formulations combine vitamin C, vitamin E, and butylated hydroxytoluene (BHT) into a product. Vitamins C and E commonly are used for both their therapeutic and formulation stability effects; BHT is used to maintain product stability.

Many types of cosmeceutical ingredient have AO properties. Highlighting the attributes of each of these ingredients is beyond the scope of this chapter. The therapeutic perspective of using enzymes, vitamins, botanical and herbal extracts, or phytochemicals for their AO potential is summarized in the subsections that follow.

Collagen [14,15]. Collagen represents up to 30% of body proteins and about 70% of dermal proteins. When it is first produced by the body, it contains high levels of water and is referred to as "soluble." As skin ages and is exposed to ultraviolet radiation, collagen loses its water, becoming more insoluble and inflexible. As a result, the skin begins to lose its texture, and wrinkles form.

Its molecular size prevents collagen from being absorbed through the skin in either soluble or insoluble form. Either type of collagen may be used in cosmeceutical products to aid product aesthetics or to give desired surface effects. The only way for collagen to aid in the repair of wrinkles, however, is via injection into the dermal layer of the skin.

Elastin [14,15]. Elastin is an insoluble protein that is present in the dermis of the skin. It gives skin the ability to retain its shape after being stressed. It is known that the amount of elastin in the skin decreases with age, causing wrinkles to appear. Elastin cannot be absorbed into the skin from cosmeceutical products because of its large molecular size.

Enzymes [16]. Enzymes are proteins that promote chemical reactions within the body and help digest food. Usually designated by the suffix "-ase," they control the reaction rates of many body processes, including the shedding of dead skin cells from the stratum corneum. Their reactivity is very dependent on pH, temperature, and the concentrations of the substrates upon which they are acting.

When the effects of a product from an enzyme reaction are not wanted, synthetic enzyme inhibitors sometimes are used. For example, the anti-tyrosinase enzyme inhibitor may aid in the lightening of skin, and the anti-elastase inhibitors stop elastin from cross-linking. The efficacy associated with using synthetic enzyme inhibitors varies with the product formulation and use conditions. More than one enzyme inhibitor can be incorporated into a multifunctional cosmeceutical product, but as discussed earlier, the physical property requirements of each active must be met.

Some enzymes require other substances for them to function. If these substances are inorganic, such as a metal ion, they are called cofactors. Cofactors may be incorporated into cosmeceuticals; however, metal ions often adversely interact with other ingredients in the formulation and can create unstable products. If the substances are complex organic molecules, such as derivatives of a vitamin, they are called coenzymes. Multifunctional cosmeceuticals often incorporate coenzymes in their formulations because they are fairly easy to formulate relative to enzymes, have better compatibility with other ingredients, and are usually less irritating to skin than many enzymes.

The proteolytic enzymes papain and bromelain have been used in cosmeceuticals to smooth or peel the skin. They must be used with extreme caution because their action is hard to stop, hence can cause severe skin irritation. Typically these actives are formulated alone or in combination with other enzymes into therapeutic cosmeceutical enzyme treatment products designed for professional use. If the enzyme formulations are too harsh to contain other cosmeceutical actives, they are often offered within a multifunctional line of cosmeceutical treatment products containing postenzyme treatments that soothe, calm, and condition the skin.

Superoxide Dismutase (SOD). A protective enzyme, SOD safeguards almost all living organisms from the damage caused by the free-radical oxygen species. Free-radical oxygen species damage cells by attacking unsaturated fatty acids in the cell membrane. In combination with the enzyme catalase, SOD completely converts these free-radical oxygen species into two water molecules plus oxygen. To further the interest in using SOD in cosmeceutical products, it is known that SOD tissue levels decrease with aging. Formulating products to contain stable SOD can be challenging, and the enzyme is irritating to skin. Modified SOD ingredients are available to aid formulation efforts.

Glycosaminoglycans [17]. Glycosaminoglycans (GAGs) are credited with maintaining the water content in skin and giving skin its elastic response. The most popular GAG used in cosmeceutical products is hyaluronic acid (HA), also called hyaluronan. A second GAG substance often used in cosmeceuticals is chondroitin. Present in both animal and human tissues at varying amounts, HA has a concentration of about 0.2 mg/mL in the human dermis. This very high molecular weight linear polymer is anionically charged at physiological pH. When HA forms hydrogen bonds, it acquires a helix structure. This helps explain its characteristic viscoelastic properties when in solution. Owing to its molecular size, HA typically is found in the basal layer of the skin, and no higher toward the skin surface than the granular layer.

It has been documented that the skin content of HA declines with age, hence the interest in using it in cosmeceutical products. Being fairly easy to incorporate into formulations, it is found in many multifunctional cosmeceutical formulations. Research has shown that HA does not penetrate through intact skin. The therapeutic benefits to having HA in products most likely are related to effects perceived at the surface of the skin.

Herbal and Botanical Extracts, and Phytochemicals [18]. Plant by-products are known to have therapeutic efficacy, hence are a major avenue for both drug discovery and cosmeceutical ingredients. A classic example of this from ancient times is the practice of chewing willow bark to alleviate pain. A major component in willow bark is salicylic acid. Salicylic acid is modified to make acetylsalicylic acid, which also is known as aspirin.

Many botanical ingredients have long histories of use from which their claims are drawn but lack documentation of their efficacy data. Because of consumer demand, the use of botanical extracts and phytochemicals in multifunctional cosmeceuticals has grown substantially. There often are several of these ingredients contained in one formula. Accordingly, it should be noted that botanical extracts are the fastest growing source of cosmeceutical allergens. A detailed discussion about specific ingredients in this category is beyond the scope of this chapter. With continued growth in documented therapeutic benefits and safety information about botanical extracts and phytochemicals, their use will also increase.

Hydroxy Acids [11,14,15,17,19–24]. A huge number of different groups of hydroxy acids exist. The groups of hydroxy acids commonly used in cosmeceuticals are α-hydroxy acids (AHAs). β-Hydroxy acids (BHAs) and α-keto acids (AKAs) also may be used. The most commonly used BHA is salicylic acid, which has been reported to yield effects similar to those of the AHAs. Enzymes may be used to effect conversion of in vivo AKAs to AHAs. The latter are also called fruit acids, reflecting their origin. For example, lactic acid is present in sour milk, honey, and tropical fruits and berries; malic acid is present in apples; citric acid is present in many fruits including oranges and lemons; glycolic and gluconic acids are present in sugarcane; and tartaric acid is present in grapes. Researchers do not completely agree on which AHA is most beneficial in cosmeceutical products; hence this discussion focuses on AHAs as a group of ingredients. Many multifunctional cosmeceuticals contain more than one type of AHA, or more than one form of an AHA.

The α-hydroxy acids have multifunctional effects on skin. They cause skin exfoliation by weakening the bonds between keratin cells and slowing cellular keratinization. They also increase the water content of skin. It has also been reported that AHAs may stimulate production of glycosaminoglycan, collagen, and elastin. Blood flow may increase to the skin tissues as a result of the dilatation of surface blood vessels. All these effects are considered beneficial to the consumer. The shedding of skin cells helps reduce the appearance of dry skin, reduces the thickness of the stratum corneum so that it looks less thick or leathery, and serves to fade spots of hyperpigmentation. The maximum therapeutic effects obtained from using AHAs usually are noted after about 2 weeks of use. As usage continues, the rate of cell renewal declines. It has been reported that the stratum corneum will remain thinner up to 2 weeks after stopping AHA product application, but overall improvements in skin changes due to AHA use may last up to 6 months.

Many of the therapeutic benefits that result from using the AHAs depend upon how they are formulated into the product. Product effects will vary with the chemical and ionic form of the acid, and with the pH of the product. Un-ionized materials penetrate the layers of the skin more readily than ionized materials. Keeping the product pH below the ionization pH keeps the AHA in an un-ionized state and enhances its ability to penetrate into the skin. Note that ionization occurs at different pH values in different AHAs. The optimum product pH depends of the objectives for product performance and the AHAs being used. Adding a buffer to the product helps keep the pH of the product constant over time. Some researchers report that amino acid salts of the AHAs yield the same therapeutic effects as pure AHAs, but with reduced skin irritation. It has also been reported that natural sources for AHAs may contain other trace substances that help reduce skin irritation. There is much controversy over these reports. Regardless of the type of AHA used and the combination of AHAs in the product, the product goal should be to deliver the desired therapeutic benefit, with minimal skin irritation.

The amount of skin exfoliation resulting from AHA use usually depends upon the type and concentration of AHA in the product. The amount of time the product is in contact with the skin and frequency of use also will greatly impact therapeutic results. Products that cause a mild exfoliation usually contain 3–6% AHA. Products designed for facial peels in a professional salon environment contain as much as 30% AHA. Products designed for chemical facial peels in a medically supervised environment contain up to 50–70% AHA. As would be expected, the higher the AHA concentration, the more irritating the product will be to the skin, and the more closely contact time with the skin must be monitored. Citric acid has been reported to be the least irritating AHA, but also is reported to have less therapeutic activity that other AHAs, even at higher concentrations. AHA products should not be used around eye, nose, and lip tissues because they are extremely irritating to delicate tissues and mucous membranes. They are commonly incorporated into multifunctional cosmeceutical products along with moisturizers, vitamins, and herbal extracts.

Lipids [25–29].   The skin's barrier layer acts to regulate the permeability of substances to and from the deeper layers of the skin, and to maintain moisture in the stratum corneum. Many factors can disrupt the function or the barrier, resulting in dry, flaky skin. Many multifunctional cosmeceutical products are targeted at maintaining or restoring barrier function. Some of these products claim to do so by impacting the lipid content of the skin. Such products typically are multifunctional and contain other ingredients, such as vitamins, herbal extracts, moisturizers, and occasionally hydroxy acids.

Lipids are essential to maintain barrier layer function. They trap water in the upper layers of the skin, and prevent water loss. Ceramides, cholesterol, and fatty acids are three of the key lipids needed to maintain barrier function. These actives often are found in combination in cosmeceutical products claiming to enhance barrier function. Note that researchers have varied opinions regarding the ability of topically applied lipids to alter the skin barrier function in dry, yet healthy, skin.

Sphingolipids are a class of lipids found throughout the skin. Ceramides are a member of the sphingolipid class. Ceramides, along with other lipoid substances, create an organized lipid network that is necessary for normal barrier function. Cosmeceutical products containing ceramides are claimed to help restore impaired skin barrier function and protect skin. They are reported to act by increasing the water-holding capacity of the stratum corneum and replacing ceramides in deficient skin. Cholesterol and fatty acids have been shown to interact with the skin's lipid network to enhance its structure and water-holding ability. Many multifunctional cosmeceutical products contain cholesterol and/or fatty acids for this reason.

Urea [30,31]. Urea is a small, soluble molecule that exists in normal skin at a concentration of about 1%. It is a component of the natural moisturizing factor (NMF), with an NMF concentration up to 7%. It functions to increase the moisture content of skin by binding to both skin proteins and water, resulting in an increase in the water content of the stratum corneum. Research shows that water both alone and with cleaning solutions decreases the amount of urea in the skin. Applying a leave-on type of urea product after washing the skin, however, can significantly increase the urea content of the skin. Urea levels may stay high as long as 24 hours or more after product application, unless the skin is washed again. Increases in skin moisture were documented to accompany the increases in skin urea levels. Urea currently is used as a moisturizer in combination with a variety of other actives in multifunctional cosmeceuticals.

Urea is inherently multifunctional from a therapeutic standpoint. This attribute stems from varied activities based on its concentration in the product. In addition to moisturizing skin, it functions to degrade keratin and to aid in the relief of itching. Since it can degrade fibrin, it is used to remove surface crusts on skin wounds. These activities occur at concentration levels of 10–30%, which can be very irritating to skin.

4.2.6 Vitamins

Vitamin A and Retinoids [1,11,14,15,23,31,33–37]. Vitamin A_1 is a fat-soluble vitamin also known as retinol. It is essential for the development and maintenance of normal skin and other tissues and bones. Once consumed, it is stored in the liver, then circulated via specific cellular binding proteins to the tissues, where it is converted to retinoic acid. Excessive vitamin A intake results in toxicity. A toxic dose of vitamin A varies with the individual, but is reported to be about 12,000 IU per kilogram of body weight. Symptoms of vitamin A toxicity can include some or all of the following: dry, peeling skin, headache, altered mental status, blurred vision, hair loss, and jaundice.

Vitamin A increases skin cell turnover. The epidermis produces more protein to become thicker, and collagen production may increase. Topically applied pure vitamin A is predominantly absorbed into the skin epidermis with only a small amount penetrating into the dermis. It is unstable in the presence of light and oxygen. When used in cosmeceutical products, vitamin A stability is poor, and it typically is inactivated within days. Since it is an oil, it often is used and classified as a skin emollient in multifunctional cosmeceutical products. Note, however, that consumers may be unaware that is serves these functions, and with a casual review of the ingredient list may think it has antiphotoaging benefits.

To enhance its stability in products, vitamin A has been chemically modified to make a variety of vitamin A esters. These esters are converted to retinol, then retinoic acid, upon absorption into the skin. The most common vitamin A ester used in multifunctional cosmeceuticals is retinyl palmitate, which is reported to be more stable than pure vitamin A. Formulation studies have been ongoing for years to understand how to keep retinyl palmitate stable for the life of a product. Its stability is affected by light, oxygen, heat, trace metals, and a product pH outside 5–6. To maintain stability, retinyl palmitate must be added to a formulation below a temperature of 40°C. Stability results have been more acceptable for products that have a stable pH between 5 and 6, contain antioxidant ingredients, and have no trace metals present. Product color stability is best for retinyl palmitate that is protected by multilamellar vesicle liposomes. Some studies indicate that retinyl palmitate penetration into the skin is enhanced when retinyl palmitate is formulated into multifunctional cosmeceutical products that also contain the AHA glycolic acid. It also has been shown that the type of product vehicle will impact the stability of retinyl palmitate, as well as its ability to penetrate into the skin.

Retinoic acid, also called tretinoin or all-*trans* retinoic acid, is available at concentrations of 0.02% to 0.1% in a emulsion, gel, or liquid vehicles via a physician's prescription. The 0.02% and 0.05% emulsion products are considered to be multifunctional cosmeceuticals because they reverse the signs of photoaging while moisturizing the skin in a fairly aesthetic cream form. They are drugs that were approved by the FDA upon completion of the NDA process. They are the only products officially indicated by the FDA for use to diminish fine wrinkles, varied skin hyperpigmentation, and skin roughness. They do not alleviate deep wrinkles, sun-damaged skin associated with cancer, coarse skin, or skin yellowing. Improvements in the indicated areas most often are perceivable after 4–6 months of use. Improvements after 6 months of use are marginal. The benefits of retinoic acid are maintained with continued product usage. Once discontinued, the skin may return to its original state. The amount of time for skin to return to its original state varies with the individual, the person's response to the product, and the amount of time that it was used. All clinical studies for 0.05% retinoic acid incorporated a complete multifunctional skin care regimen that included sunscreens and protective clothing.

Retinoic acid is a known skin irritant and causes photosensitivity. The degree of side effects associated with retinoic acid use vary, but most often include skin redness, itching, burning, stinging, peeling, and dryness. Symptoms typically subside within 6 months of continued use. Patients may opt to reduce the frequency of product application to manage skin reactions. About 4% of patients discontinue retinoic acid use because of their inability to tolerate adverse skin reactions. Retinoic acid use is not recommended during pregnancy.

Vitamin B [32,38].   There are many different types of vitamin B, and their functions are not the same. The two types of vitamin B used most often in multifunctional cosmeceuticals are β-carotene and panthenol. Different types of vitamin B commonly are combined a multifunctional cosmeceutical product.

β-Carotene, found in carrot oil, acts predominantly as an antioxidant. When consumed in the diet, it is transformed by the body into vitamin A. Product formulation with β-carotene is challenging because it stains the skin yellow. Decolorizing β-carotene so that it will not stain the skin often results in the loss of its therapeutic activity.

Panthenol is active in the form called D-panthenol. It is found naturally in liver, queen bee jelly, rice bran, and molasses. It is absorbed after topical application, and converted in the skin to D-panthenoic acid. D-Panthenoic acid works with skin enzymes to enhance skin cell growth and promote skin healing. D-Panthenol also is classified as a moisturizer in cosmeceutical products.

Vitamin C [11,15,23,32,38–40].   Vitamin C also is known as L-ascorbic acid. It is found in citrus fruits, hip berries, fresh tea leaves, and paprika. Vitamin C is therapeutically multifunctional in that it is recognized as an antioxidant and functions as a cofactor that is necessary for many in vivo reactions to occur. It facilitates collagen production in tissue cells, reduces the likelihood of infection in wounds, and converts reacted vitamin E back into its active form, restoring the capacity of vitamin E to function as a free-radical scavenger. The L-ascorbic acid isomer of vitamin C can be absorbed after topical application and has been shown to reduce the amount of ultraviolet photodamage to skin cells. It is documented to act in concert with other skin antioxidants to yield this benefit. Vitamin C also has been reported to stimulate skin collagen production under certain conditions. Research continues to examine the extent of these effects on healthy, intact human skin.

Since vitamin C is such a good antioxidant, it is difficult to keep stable in a formulation. Stable formulations that contain 10% L-ascorbic acid in an acidic aqueous form are available, but significant clinical data demonstrating their antiphotoaging benefits are lacking. Research also is investigating the usefulness of vitamin C derivatives. Ascorbyl palmitate and phosphate are contained in many multifunctional cosmeceutical products. These esters are easier to formulate into products than L-ascorbic acid, but more research in needed to document their ability to penetrate the human stratum corneum to produce a therapeutic effect.

Vitamin E [11,15,32,41,42]. Vitamin E is a fat-soluble vitamin, which in its most potent form is known as α-tocopherol. It has multifunctional benefits. It most commonly is used in multifunctional cosmeceutical products as a moisturizer, and as a stabilizer for other ingredients against oxidation. Research shows that vitamin E has additional benefits for the skin: it is necessary to stabilize cell membranes; it is thought to control parameters impacting the structure and function of various lipoproteins; and its antioxidant effects are thought to be protective against substances that may have damaging effects on the skin. Its free-radical scavenging activity makes for its photoprotective effects against ultraviolet radiation. Research indicates that the application of topical vitamin E can result in increased vitamin E content in the epidermis for at least 24 hours. It enhances the ability of other antioxidants within the skin to protect skin tissues, and is noted to stop ultraviolet-induced immunosupression and tumorigenesis. Vitamin E has been noted to reduce the incidence of various skin irritations. Caution must be exercised, however, because some topical products containing 10–20% vitamin E have been reported to irritate the skin, resulting in delayed eczema or rash-type reactions.

Vitamin E stability is compromised by heat, light, and the presence of metal ions. Its oxidation is relatively slow, however, thus allowing its widespread use in many multifunctional cosmeceutical products. Vitamin E can be modified into an ester form, and the most popular ester used in cosmeceuticals is vitamin E acetate, a compound that is very stable against oxidation. When orally ingested, vitamin E acetate is transformed into vitamin E. The same conversion must be made in the skin after topical application to yield vitamin E benefits, but studies have not definitively confirmed this conversion. Understanding more about the penetration of vitamin E acetate into the skin, and the rate at which it is converted into vitamin E, will shed more light on the potential value of using this ester instead of vitamin E. Vitamin E acetate is not thought to be photoprotective.

Pure α-tocopherol rarely exists in nature, but it is commercially produced and available. Natural vitamin E, a mixture of different forms of vitamin E, is present in wheat germ, corn, sunflower seeds, grape seeds, soybean oils, alfalfa, and lettuce.

4.3 Choosing Excipients

"Excipient" is a term used to describe the portion of a formulation that does not include the actives [9]. There are many excipient ingredients available from which to choose, and many of them have inherent multifunctional character. For example, glycerin may act as a skin moisturizer as well as a product humectant. To efficiently create a product, excipients should be chosen based on their intended function in the product, and their physical and chemical properties. The formulation must be created around the needs of the identified actives. Ideally, the excipients should enhance the ability of the actives to render their therapeutic benefits, as well as contribute to the multifunctional nature of the product. Changing the concentration of excipients in a cosmeceutical formulation can alter the performance of the actives. In addition, substituting excipient ingredients, even though the ingredients may be thought to be similar in nature, can alter the performance of the actives. Any excipient changes in a product should be followed with studies that confirm the function of the actives in the new formula.

A major consideration in the choice of excipients is final product stability. The goal is to build a product that will, at a minimum, remain unchanged until the consumer is through using it. This is typically considered to be at least 2 years from the time of production. Since excipients are elective ingredients, choosing ones that have predictable stability profiles will afford more time to address other development issues. Note that different package types can influence the stability of excipients and actives alike. Different package sizes and components allow various degrees of product exposure to air, light, and moisture. If possible, choose excipients based on their performance in the package type intended for the product.

Some excipients may contribute to skin or eye irritation. As with actives, the irritation potential of an excipient may vary with the excipient form that is used. Owing to the vast number of excipient ingredients to choose from, it is best to avoid ones that are likely to contribute to an unwanted product issue, particularly if potentially irritating actives are required. If potentially irritating excipients are essential to the formulation, their content should be kept to a minimum. Depending upon the type of irritation associated with the excipients, other ingredients may be available that can help counteract the excipient irritation. As with actives, there may be differences between excipient production lots and excipient manufacturers. Evaluation standards should be established for each excipient before approval is granted for use in a product.

Multifunctional cosmeceutical products must meet or exceed the aesthetic expectations of the consumer. Typically, it is the combination of excipients that determines the aesthetic character of a formulation. Choosing ingredients that contribute to good product aesthetics while serving their intended function makes good formulation sense. The classifications of excipients often found in many multifunctional cosmeceutical products include surfactants, emulsifiers, stabilizers, thickeners, water, alcohols, humectants, triglycerides, fatty acids, oils, extracts, waxes, semisolids, silicones, preservatives, antioxidants, and fragrances.

4.4   Developing the Product Vehicle

In the pharmaceutical industry, the product vehicle is often referred to as the active delivery system. In essence, multifunctional cosmeceuticals offer consumers an aesthetic active delivery system. As with pharmaceutical products, vehicles are known to change product efficacy. The challenge in formulating multifunctional cosmeceutical products is to maintain active efficacies, while creating aesthetic vehicles. Note that product viscosity and application technique also impact the active efficacy. Knowing how the consumer will use the product, and how the product will be dispensed from the package, can aid in creating formulations that maximize the therapeutic benefits of actives.

After the properties of the actives have been carefully considered, and excipients thoughtfully chosen, the best procedure for preparing the product must be determined. Different methods of preparing products often produce varied aesthetic and stability results, with varied active efficacies. When one is uncertain about the best approach to compounding a formulation, alternate approaches should be tried. Accelerated stability protocol must be used to screen the prototype products. Once prototype stability has been confirmed, then verification of the active and product performance must be confirmed.

5   CONCLUSION

Regardless of the term chosen, or the regulations to follow, multifunctional "cosmeceutical" products are an essential part of the cosmetic and toiletry market. Their development and use will increase in coming years. The key to preserving the multifunctional character of cosmeceutical products is to take the time to obtain all the essential information about the actives and product excipients before starting formulation. This information should be used to develop a formulation plan. Initial formulations should be very simple, and built around the actives to ensure active efficacy. When one is creating or evaluating any multifunctional cosmeceutical product, it is important to assess the following parameters [15]:

1. The actives present in the product are in forms that the skin can use to achieve the claimed benefits.
2. The actives present in the product are at a high enough concentration to render a benefit after product application under normal use conditions, and for expected skin sites and types.
3. The actives present in the product are stable in the product for as long as the consumer is expected to take to finish it.
4. The delivery system chosen for the actives, and the recommended use conditions, allow the actives to be delivered in a manner that will yield therapeutic benefits. For example, will a wash-off or a leave-on type of product better allow the active to render its therapeutic benefits?

5. The benefits expected from reading the multifunctional cosmeceutical product claims are realized with product usage, and the product will perform as intended for the expected life of the product.

REFERENCES

1. SH McNamara. FDA regulation of cosmeceuticals. Cosmet Toiletries 112(3):41–45, 1997.
2. W Umbach. Cosmeceuticals—The future of cosmetics? Cosmet Toiletries 110(11): 33–40, 1995.
3. H Epstein. Factors in formulating cosmeceutical vehicles. Cosmet Toiletries 112(10): 91–99, 1997.
4. AM Kligman. Why cosmeceuticals? Cosmet Toiletries 108(8):37–38, 1993.
5. AM Kligman. Cosmeceuticals as a third category. Cosmet Toiletries 113(2):33–40, 1998.
6. A Osol, ed. Remington's Pharmaceutical Sciences. 16th ed. Easton, PA: Mack Publishing, 1980.
7. HC Ansel, NG Popovich. Pharmaceutical Dosage Forms and Drug Delivery Systems. 5th ed. Philadelphia: Lea & Febiger, 1990.
8. P Frost, SN Horwitz. Principles of Cosmetics for the Dermatologist. St. Louis, MD: CV Mosby, 1982.
9. BL Radd. Efficient formulation of cosmeceutical products. Cosmet Toiletries 109(10):51–56, 1994.
10. A Martin, J Swarbrick, A Cammarata. Physical Pharmacy: Physical Chemical Principles in the Pharmaceutical Sciences. 3rd ed. Philadelphia: Lea & Febiger, 1983.
11. S Budavari, ed. The Merck Index. 12th ed. Whitehouse Station, NJ: Merck 1996.
12. JL Zatz. Optimizing skin delivery. Cosmet Toiletries 115(1):31–56, 2000.
13. JW Wiechers. Avoiding transdermal cosmetic delivery. Cosmet Toiletries 115(2):39–46, 2000.
14. R Hermitte. Aged skin, retinoids and alpha hydroxy acids. Cosmet Toiletries 107(7): 63–67, 1992.
15. BL Radd. Anitwrinkle ingredients. Skin Inc 9(1):88–99, 1997.
16. G Brooks, DB Scholz, D Parish, S Bennett. Aging and the future of enzymes in cosmetics. Cosmet Toiletries 112(11):79–89, 1997.
17. MG Tucci, MM Belmonte, G Biagini, E Vellucci, P Morganti, O Talassi, R Solmi, G Ricotta. AHAs and derivatives. Cosmet Toiletries 113(3):55–58, 1998.
18. D Steinberg. Frequency used of botanicals. Cosmet Toiletries 113(10):73–77, 1998.
19. WP Smith. Hydroxy acids and skin aging. Cosmet Toiletries 109(9):41–88, 1994.
20. HH Roenigk. Treatment of the aging face. Dermatol Clin 13(2):246–261, 1995.
21. MG Rubin. Therapeutics: Personal practice, the clinical use of alpha hydroxy acids. Austral J Dermatol 35:29–33, 1994.
22. R Scheinberg. Alpha hydroxy acids for skin rejuvenation. West J Med 160(4): 366–367, 1994.
23. AB Lewis, EC Gendler. Resurfacing with topical agents. Semin Cutan Med Surg 15(3):139–144, 1996.

24. A Sah, S Mukherjee, RR Wickett. An in vitro study of the effects of formulation variables and product structure on percutaneous absorption of lactic acid. J Soc Cosmet Chem 49(4):257–273, 1998.

25. M Rieger. Ceramides: Their promise in skin care. Cosmet Toiletries 111(12):33–45, 1996.

26. M Pauly, G Pauly. Glycoderamides. Cosmet Toiletries 110(8):49–56, 1995.

27. RS Summers, B Summers, P Chandar, C Feinberg, R Gursky, AV Rawlings. The effect of lipids, with and without humcetant, on skin xerosis. J Soc Cosmet Chem 47(1):27–39, 1996.

28. M Mao-Qiang, KR Feingold, F Wang, CR Thornfeldt, PM Elias. A natural lipid mixture improves barrier function and hydration in human and murine skin. J Soc Cosmet Chem 47(3):157–166, 1996.

29. AV Rawlings, A Watkinson, CR Harding, C Ackerman, J Banks, J Hope, R Scott. Changes in stratum corneum lipid and desmosome structure together with water barrier function during mechanical stress. J Soc Cosmet Chem 46(3):141–151, 1995.

30. D Hantschel, G Sauermann, H Steinhart, U Hoppe, J Ennen. Urea analysis of extracts from stratum corneum and the role of urea-supplemented cosmetics. J Soc Cosmet Chem 49(3):155–163, 1998.

31. TH Burnham, ed. Drug Facts and Comparisons. St. Louis, MD: Facts and Comparisons, 2000.

32. B Idson. Vitamins and the skin. Cosmet Toiletries 108(12):79–94, 1993.

33. PM Campos, GM Eccleston. Vitamin A skin penetration. Cosmet Toiletries 113(7): 69–72, 1998.

34. HG Ji, BS Seo. Retinyl palmitate at 5% in a cream: Its stability, efficacy and effect. Cosmet Toiletries 114(3):61–68, 1999.

35. GR Leonardi, PM Campos. Influence of glycolic acid as a component of different formulations on skin penetration by vitamin A palmitate. J Soc Cosmet Chem 49(1):23–32, 1998.

36. PM Campos, G Ricci, M Semprini, R Lopes. Histopathological, morphometric, and stereologic studies of dermocosmetic skin formulations containing vitamin A and/or glycolic acid. J Soc Cosmet Chem 50(3):159–170, 1999.

37. KR Olson, ed. Poisoning & Drug Overdose. 2nd ed. Norwalk, CT: Appleton & Lange, 1994.

38. WP Smith, D Mae, K Marenus, L Calvo. Natural cosmetic ingredients: Enhanced function. Cosmet Toiletries 106(2):65–71, 1991.

39. MR Silva, DML Contente, A Oliveira, PA Filho. Ascorbic acid liberation from O/W/O multiple emulsions. Cosmet Toiletries 112(12):85–87, 1997.

40. RM Colven, SR Pinnell. Topical vitamin C in aging. Clin Dermatol 14:227–234, 1996.

41. D Billek. Cosmetics for elderly people. Cosmet Toiletries 111(7):31–37, 1996.

42. M Rangarajan, JL Zatz. Skin delivery of vitamin E. J Soc Cosmet Chem 50(4):249–279, 1999.

8

Multifunctional Oral Care Products

M. J. Tenerelli
Upland Editorial, East Northport, New York, U.S.A.

There was a time when toothpaste cleaned your teeth and mouthwash freshened your breath, and that was that. Not anymore. Today, oral care products promise at least two, if not three or four, different ways to bolster your oral health and beautify your face. Toothpastes that clean also battle gum disease and turn pearly whites whiter. Mouthwash fights plaque as well as halitosis. These innovations in oral care products are a direct response to the busy modern consumer, who wants one product to do effectively as many things as possible. While toothpastes and mouthwash share some basic ingredients, the special extra functions they endeavor to provide call for different and specific ingredients for each formulation.

1 TECHNOLOGY OF INCORPORATING SPECIAL INGREDIENTS

An important aspect of creating multifunctional oral care products is the incorporation of active ingredients. The usual toothpaste ingredients used must be formulated so that they do not interfere with the activity of special ingredients. Take fluoride, for example, which is found in most toothpastes. The formulator must be careful that the cavity-fighting properties of the fluoride are not compromised by the introduction of a special ingredient, say a bleach or abrasive, to make a whitening toothpaste. Sodium monofluorophosphate works well with both silica and calcium abrasives, while the ideal abrasive to incorporate with sodium fluoride is silica. Because there is no chemical interaction between sodium fluoride and the silica abrasive, the fluoride is free to be released in saliva during brushing, instead of becoming trapped in the surface of the abrasive. Consider also the following scenario. To make toothpastes effective in the fight against gingivitis, or gum disease, the antibacterial agent triclosan is now added to a regular toothpaste formulation. However, the kind of surfactant used in a toothpaste for foaming may hamper the delivery system for the triclosan. To avoid compromising the effectiveness of the triclosan, formulators choose the anionic surfactant sodium lauryl sulfate, as opposed to an nonionic surfactant, which could adhere strongly enough to triclosan to immobilize its effect on the gums.

Ingredients added to oral care products to make them multifunctional are usually not inert and require careful selection of compatible toothpaste or mouthwash components. The product, on top of that, must still taste good and possess the top shelf physical properties to which the customer is accustomed. Preparing such oral care products requires formulation experience and a strong education in the physicochemical properties of the raw materials, surface and colloid chemistry, and rheology.

2 TOOTHPASTE

All toothpastes share some basic ingredients: mild detergents and abrasives, as well as fluoride. Humectants, binders, thickeners, flavoring and coloring agents, preservatives, and sweeteners are also standard components of toothpaste formulations. From there the ingredient list will vary considerably, depending on the functions (aside from basic cleaning) that the product is meant to provide.

Common basic toothpaste ingredients include the following:

> *Detergents:* sodium lauryl sulfate, cocoamidopropyl betaine
> *Fluoride:* sodium monofluorophosphate, stannous fluoride, sodium fluoride
> *Abrasives:* dicalcium phosphate dihydrate, insoluble sodium metaphosphate, calcium pyrophosphate, calcium carbonate, alumina trihydrate, magnesium trisilicate, silica gels
> *Humectants:* glycerol, sorbitol
> *Binders:* natural gums, seaweed colloids, synthetic celluloses
> *Flavors:* generally, peppermint, spearmint, and wintergreen, modified with other essential oils such as cinnamon, menthol, and eucalyptus.
> *Colors:* titanium dioxide for white pastes; various food dyes for colored pastes and gels

2.1 Whitening Toothpaste

Over-the-counter (OTC) toothpastes that strive to bring a whiter shade of pale to your teeth are often labeled "advanced whitening formulas." These products do not increase the whiteness of the underlying tooth. Instead, they remove or fade stains so that the underlying whiteness of the tooth becomes more visible. There are several ways manufacturers accomplish this. One way is through the use of abrasives to "polish" away stains and discolorations. Another way is through the use of bleaching agents, such as peroxide. Some brands incorporate enzymes to remove stains.

The degree of whitening achieved will depend on the percentage of bleaching agent or abrasive included in the toothpaste, as well as the type of abrasive used. Hydrogen peroxide and carbamide peroxide are the two bleaching agents usually present in OTC whitening toothpastes. Abrasives commonly found in whitening toothpaste are the same as those found in regular toothpaste, although the abrasive concentration may be higher. Sodium pyrophospate is an example of a powerful abrasive found in advanced whitening toothpaste formulas.

New innovations in OTC whitening products for teeth include at-home bleaching kits, which contain trays and a bleaching agent to be left on for several hours at a time or overnight, and peroxide-infused whitening strips, which are placed against the teeth and left in place for approximately 30 minutes at a time, over a period of approximately 2 weeks. The peroxide levels in these products are higher than those found in OTC whitening toothpastes.

2.2 Toothpaste for Sensitive Teeth

Some toothpaste are meant to help prevent pain in teeth sensitive to heat, cold, and pressure. Sensitive teeth are usually the result of recession of the gums, which has led to expose tooth roots. Because the roots are not protected by enamel, the small channels leading to the pulp of the tooth are vulnerable to environmental factors like heat and cold.

Toothpaste formulations geared for sensitive teeth work by either deadening nerve endings or making teeth less porous. Active ingredients commonly used to block access to the tooth root include fluoride and either potassium nitrate or strontium chloride.

Most toothpastes for sensitive teeth contain about 5% potassium nitrate or strontium chloride. The ingredients work with minerals present in saliva to crystallize and cover the pores in teeth, blocking entry to the roots. Results should be apparent after several weeks of using an OTC toothpaste for sensitive teeth.

2.3 Tartar Control Toothpaste

Tartar control toothpastes help prevent the formation of tartar (which can lead to gum disease). When mixed with minerals in saliva, plaque hardens into the white or yellowish deposit called tartar. The active ingredient in tartar control toothpastes are primarily pyrophosphates. These work by clinging to the teeth above the gum line and absorbing the plaque that would otherwise collect on teeth and harden.

Tartar control toothpaste cannot remove tartar once it has formed. Only professional cleaning can do that.

The pyrophosphates in tartar control toothpastes exhibit the following beneficial actions:

Disrupt the crystalline structure of plaque
Regulate the percentage of calcium in saliva
Become absorbed into tooth enamel as a calcium complex
Discourage the formation of tartar through calcium-infused lattice attached
    to enamel

2.4 Toothpaste That Targets Gingivitis

As of 2002, only one toothpaste on the U.S. market has been allowed by the U.S. Food and Drug Administration to claim antigingivitis properties. The toothpaste, a multicare product that is meant to fight plaque and cavities as well as gingivitis, targets the gum disease with a combination of sodium fluoride, triclosan, and a copolymer.

Triclosan is an antibacterial agent often found in soaps and deodorants. As an ingredient in toothpaste, it inhibits the growth of bacteria in plaque. Bacteria in plaque can produce harmful acids, toxins, and enzymes that damage surrounding gum tissues. The redness, swelling, tenderness, and bleeding of gums that result from plaque buildup are the symptoms of gingivitis.

The copolymer Gantrez™ extends the life of the triclosan so that it remains on teeth and gums for approximately 12 hours after brushing, giving long-life protection against gingivitis.

2.5 Baking Soda Toothpaste

Baking soda in toothpaste is a type of whitener, meant to work as a low level abrasive that cleanses and removes stains on teeth. It is often added to a formulation because consumers enjoy the freshness it imparts to the mouth. It is often added in combination with peroxide in a toothpaste to provide a bubbling, clean-tasting action between teeth and in other hard-to-reach areas.

Baking sodas commonly found in toothpaste include sodium bicarbonate (bicarbonate of soda), sodium hydrogen carbonate, and sodium acid carbonate.

2.6 Toothpaste with Mouthwash

Several toothpastes are available now that purport not only to cleanse and fight cavities but to more powerfully freshen breath through the addition of OTC mouthwash. Mouthwash formulations are discussed later in the chapter. When mouthwash is added to toothpaste, the formulator must once again be careful that the mouthwash itself does not interfere with the working of other ingredients within a toothpaste.

2.7   Multitudes of Multicare Toothpastes

An abundance of multifunctional toothpastes is available on today's OTC market. The preceding sections described toothpastes that cleanse and perform one other function. Following are types of toothpaste that perform two, three, or more functions on top of cleansing:

> Whitening/tartar control/anticavity
> Whitening/tartar control/anticavity/breath freshener
> Whitening/tartar control/gingivitis protection/anticavity
> Whitening/tartar control/gingivitis protection/anticavity/breath freshener
> Sensitive tooth care/anticavity
> Sensitive tooth care/anticavity/whitening
> Sensitive tooth care/anticavity/tartar control

3   MOUTHWASH

Mouthwash works in several different ways to fight bad breath. One way is to reduce the number of anaerobic bacteria in a person's mouth. These bacteria produce the volatile sulfur compounds that are the actual cause of halitosis. In other words, the mouthwash kills the bad germs that cause bad breath.

Mouthwash can also be formulated to neutralize volatile sulfur compounds already formed. Finally, it can work by masking the bad breath with a stronger and pleasanter scent, like peppermint or cinnamon.

Chlorine dioxide is an active ingredient common to many OTC mouthwash products. It both reduces anaerobic bacteria and neutralizes volatile sulfur compounds. Chlorine dioxide come in regular and stable forms. Most manufacturers use stabilized chlorine dioxide for its superior staying power within a solution. When adding chlorine dioxide to a mouthwash solution, formulators need to be careful not to mix the ingredient with a flavoring agent like peppermint or spearmint. This is because chlorine dioxide reacts with organic compounds, including flavoring agents, which means that the additive will react with flavoring agents, if present, instead of fighting halitosis.

Another ingredient found in some popular mouthwash is zinc. This mineral works to neutralize volatile sulfur compounds. It is thought that zinc ions bind to the precursor compounds used by anaerobic bacteria to create volatile sulfur compounds, inhibiting their creation.

Antiseptic mouthwashes, extremely popular with consumers today, do double duty, cleaning the breath and protecting the mouth. They work by killing off oral anaerobic bacteria. Their purpose is to help prevent cavities and gingivitis.

The active ingredients that can provide this action in OTC mouthwashes include alcohol, cetylpyridinium chloride, menthol, eucalyptol, thymol, and methyl salicylate.

Today mouthwashes endeavor to do a number of good things for your mouth as well as your breath. They are touted as preventing and fighting tartar, preventing and reducing plaque, and preventing and reducing gingivitis, as well as fighting bad breath.

3.1 Fluoride Rinses

Some mouthwashes contain fluoride to help battle tooth decay by hardening the enamel surface of the teeth.

3.2 Antiplaque Rinses

Antiplaque rinses can contain active ingredients meant to help loosen and remove plaque from teeth and the gum line. These ingredients can include phenol, metal salts, and a botanical such as sanguinaria.

4 CONCLUSION

A convergence between consumer demand and increasing technological sophistication has led to oral care products that can do a number of things all at once: cleanse, whiten, soothe, and freshen; inhibit plaque growth and help remove it; prevent gum disease; and block exposed nerves and fend off cavities. A whole new way of formulating oral care products is now at hand. To do the category justice, today's creators of oral care products must be well versed in the physicochemical properties of the raw materials, surface and colloid chemistry, and rheology.

9

Sun Protectants: Enhancing Product Functionality with Sunscreens

Joseph W. Stanfield
Suncare Research Laboratories, LLC, Memphis, Tennessee, U.S.A.

1 INTRODUCTION

The effective use of sunscreens to enhance cosmetic functionality requires an understanding of the need for sunscreen protection in terms of the solar radiation environment and current knowledge of the damaging effects of sunlight on human skin. In addition, the number of available active ingredients is limited, and procedures for sunscreen performance evaluations are complex. The currently nebulous restrictions on sunscreen label claims present challenges in formulating combination products. The purpose of this chapter is to provide an understanding of the state of the art of sun protection to facilitate development of innovative multifunctional products incorporating sun protective ingredients.

2 THE SOLAR ULTRAVIOLET SPECTRUM

The ultraviolet (UV) spectrum of sunlight contains significant amounts of energy over the wavelength range from approximately 300 to 400 nm, which is the thresh-

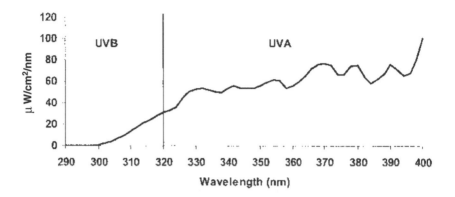

FIGURE 1   The standard solar spectrum. (From Ref. 2.)

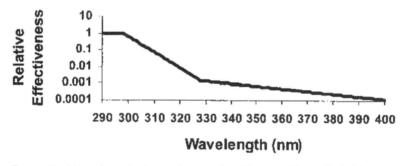

FIGURE 2   Wavelength dependence of erythema. (From Ref. 4.)

old of violet light [1]. The Solar UV spectrum is divided into the UVA region, from 320 to 400 nm, and the UVB region, from 290 to 320 nm. The "standard" solar spectrum published by COLIPA, (the European Cosmetic, Toiletry, and Perfumery Association (Fig. 1), represents a midsummer, noon, mid latitude solar UV spectrum [2].

Energy from the UV wavelengths in sunlight produces the signs and symptoms of human sunburn, including redness, pain, blistering, swelling, and eventually peeling of the skin—in the most extreme cases. Erythema is the "redness" component of sunburn [3,4]. Energy in the UV wavelengths has also been shown to produce skin cancer [5], as well as skin changes associated with photoaging [6] in mice and changes in the skin immune response in mice [7] and humans [8]. The shorter UVB wavelengths (290–320 nm) are more effective in producing virtually all forms of UV damage than the longer UVA wavelengths (320–400 nm), but since the solar UV spectrum contains at least 10-fold more UVA power than UVB power, even the former contributes substantially to these effects [3–5,7,8].

The McKinlay–Diffey action spectrum (wavelength dependence relationship) for erythema (Fig. 2) illustrates that UV energy with a wavelength of 400 nm is only about one ten-thousandth as effective in producing sunburn as UV energy with a wavelength of 290 nm [4].

3 SUNSCREEN INGREDIENTS

Sunscreen ingredients are chemicals that absorb and/or scatter incident radiation, thus attenuating ultraviolet energy before it can penetrate the skin. The U.S. Food and Drug Administration (FDA) lists 16 chemicals approved for use as active ingredients in sunscreen products (Table 1) [9]. Since each active ingredient, depending on its chemical structure, absorbs energy in a limited region of the solar UV spectrum, most sunscreen products contain a combination of two or more

Table 1 Active Ingredients and Maximum Permissible Concentrations Approved for Use In Sunscreen Products

Ingredient	Maximum permissible concentration (%)
Aminobenzoic acid	15
Avobenzone	3
Cinoxate	3
Dioxybenzone	3
Homosalate	15
Menthyl anthranilate	5
Octocrylene	10
Octyl methoxycinnamate	7.5
Octyl salicylate	5
Oxybenzone	6
Padimate O	8
Phenylbenzimidazolesulfonic acid	4
Sulisobenzone	10
Titanium dioxide	25
Trolamine salicylate	12
Zinc oxide	25

Source: Ref. 9.

active ingredients. For example, a popular sunscreen ingredient, approved by the FDA in 1978 as ethylhexyl *p*-methoxycinnamate [10] and now known as Octinoxate [11], absorbs maximally at a wavelength of about 305 nm, in the UVB region. A newer, more recently approved sunscreen ingredient, Avobenzone, absorbs maximally at 355 nm, in the UVA region [9,12]. To ensure absorption of energy across the entire solar UV spectrum, a typical modern sunscreen product might contain a combination of these two ingredients.

4   SUN PROTECTION FACTOR (SPF)

The degree to which a sunscreen product protects against sunburn (erythema) is described by the sun protection factor (SPF). The SPF is the ratio of the minimal erythema dose (MED) on human skin protected by a sunscreen to the MED without a sunscreen present. In the SPF test prescribed by the FDA [9], the MED is determined by administering a series of progressively increasing UV energy doses and evaluating the responses 22–24 later. The MED is the smallest dose of UV energy that produces erythema with distinct borders in the exposure site. For labeling purposes, the SPF of a sunscreen product is the next lowest whole number below the mean SPF, for a panel of at least 20 qualified human volunteer subjects, less the 95% confidence interval. Although the FDA Sunscreen Monograph [9] specifies an upper limit of 30 (or 30+) on labeled SPF, marketed sunscreen products currently have labeled SPF values ranging from 2 to at least 60. Vaughan et al. have recently shown that sun bathers may be exposed to more than 30 MEDs in a single day at the beach in South Florida [13].

The SPF is the ratio of protected MED to unprotected MED. Another way of thinking of SPF is as the reciprocal of the transmission of sunburning energy, T. Thus

$$\text{SPF} = \frac{1}{T} \tag{9.1}$$

Therefore a sunscreen with an SPF of 2 transmits 50% of the sunburning energy it receives, an SPF of 15 transmits 6.7%, and a sunscreen with an SPF of 30 transmits 3.3%. A sunscreen with an SPF of 50 would still transmit 2%. This illustrates the diminishing benefits of increasing SPF values.

The spectral distribution of sunscreen UV protection is visualized by plotting the thin-film absorbance spectrum of the sunscreen against wavelength. The thin-film absorbance spectrum may be obtained by applying a thin film of sunscreen to a suitable substrate and using a spectroradiometer to measure the UV transmission at each wavelength. The absorbance at each wavelength is calculated as follows:

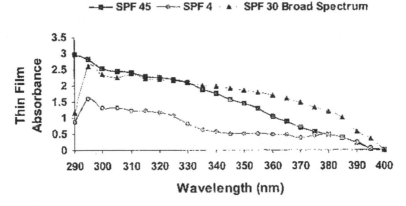

FIGURE 3 Sunscreen absorbance spectra.

$$A = -\log(\text{transmission}) \tag{9.2}$$

Thin-film absorbance spectra are shown in Figure 3 for sunscreen products with SPF values of 4, 30, and 45. The SPF 30 product contains Avobenzone and is considered to be a broad-spectrum sunscreen. It is apparent from Figure 3 that the SPF 30 and 45 products have higher absorbance values than the SPF 4 product over the entire UV spectrum. The SPF 45 product has higher UV absorbance at the shorter, more erythemally effective UVB wavelengths than the SPF 30 product, but the SPF 30 product has higher absorbance in the UVA region.

Since SPF is a measure of sunscreen protection against erythema in humans, and since erythema is predominantly caused by UVB wavelengths, SPF is primarily a measure of UVB protection. The action spectra for nonmelanoma skin cancer and UV-induced skin elastosis in mice are similar to the action spectra for erythema [5,6]. Although the link between human malignant melanoma and UV exposure is not well understood, recent studies suggest that UVB is more important than UVA in that condition, as well [14,15]. In addition, a recent study in humans by Naylor et al. in the United States [16] and another by Thompson et al. in Australia [17] demonstrated that sunscreen use during sun exposure may reduce the development of actinic keratoses, which are believed to be precancerous lesions [18].

Two concerns about sunscreen protection are product removal by swimming and sweating and use of the proper application amount by consumers. The FDA Final Sunscreen Monograph contains a procedure for measuring SPF after 40 or 80 min of water immersion. If the labeled SPF is measured without water immersion, it is referred to as the "static" SPF. If the labeled SPF is based on the 40 or

80 min test, the sunscreen product may be labeled as "water resistant" or "very water resistant" [9], respectively. The SPF test requires application of product at 2 mg/cm^2 [9]. Thus to realize the labeled SPF, consumers must be instructed to apply the same amount of product per unit area that was used for measuring the label SPF. This translates to approximately 40 g of product per application for full-body coverage for an average adult consumer, or only three to four applications per 4-ounce bottle.

5   UVA PROTECTION

5.1   Effects of UVA

Data from animal studies suggest that sunscreens prevent development of skin cancer, and that UVA protection may be as important as UVB protection in that respect [18]. As noted earlier, energy in the UV wavelengths has also been shown to cause changes in the skin immune response. Moyal, who evaluated the level of protection by two broad-spectrum sunscreens with the same SPF, but with differ-ent UVA protection factors, against acute solar-simulated UV radiation-induced immunosuppression in humans, found that the sunscreen with the higher UVA protection factor was substantially more protective [8]. Perhaps the most impor-tant reason for the need for high levels of UVA protection is that SPF is determined by using solar simulators that typically lack the relative levels of UVA power found in sunlight at most latitudes and may overestimate the degree of sun pro-tection actually received [19]. Calculations made by using solar spectra and sun-screen transmission spectra show that products providing high levels of UVA pro-tection are more protective than products with similar labeled SPFs for the solar spectra most frequently encountered by consumers.

Increasing awareness of the need for skin protection against the UVA por-tion of the solar spectrum (320–400 nm) has accelerated development of sun-screen products that provide substantial UVA protection. Since these products have labeled SPF values similar to those of products that provide primarily UVB protection and relatively little UVA protection, there is a need for a reliable and informative index of UVA protection.

5.2   Measuring UVA Protection

The assessment of UVA protection is a formidable problem, because sunlight is always a mixture of UVA and UVB, and the immediate and long-term effects of UVA are normally masked by the effects of energy in the more potent UVB wave-lengths. Separation of UVA effects from those of full-spectrum UV is difficult, and eliciting measurable responses to UVA alone requires high energy doses and rel-atively long exposure times.

Proposed human in vivo methods for assessing UVA protection include the immediate pigment darkening (IPD) method, the persistent pigment darkening (PPD) method, and the protection factor A (PFA) method. While each has its advantages, none is completely adequate for assigning a clinically relevant index of sunscreen protection in the UVA region.

5.2.1 Immediate Pigment Darkening

The immediate pigment darkening (IPD) response is a transient brownish-gray coloration of the skin of individuals with pigmented skin after irradiation with UVA radiation. The response is evaluated within 60 s after UVA exposure. The IPD protection factor, proposed by Kaidbey and Barnes, is the ratio of the UVA dose required to produce the response, with and without a sunscreen on the skin [20].

The IPD test produces rapid results with low doses of UVA. However the response is highly variable and difficult to reproduce accurately. Its clinical significance is low because the action spectrum for IPD differs widely from action spectra for erythema and tanning [3,4,21], nonmelanoma skin cancer [5], and photoelastosis [6]. Further, the test is performed using human subjects with skin types III and IV, who are less sun sensitive than types I and II and are not the individuals who have the greatest need for sun protection. (The sun-reactive skin types were characterized by Fitzpatrick [22].) In addition, the low UVA doses involved may conceal the effects of sunlight on the photostability of the product (see later).

5.2.2 Persistent Pigment Darkening

The persistent pigment darkening (PPD) response is a longer lasting response of individuals with pigmented skin after irradiation with UVA radiation. The response is evaluated 2–24 h after UVA exposure. The PPD protection factor, proposed by Chardon et al. [23], is the ratio of the UVA dose required to produce the PPD response, with and without a sunscreen on the skin.

The PPD test produces rapid results with moderately low doses of UVA. The response is stable and reproducible; as in the case of IPD, however, its clinical significance is low because the action spectrum for PPD is not defined for wavelengths shorter than 320 nm. Further, the test is performed on human subjects with skin types II, III, and IV, whereas type I individuals are the most sun sensitive, hence have the greatest need for sun protection.

5.2.3 PFA

The PFA (protection factor A) method, proposed by Cole and Van Fossen [24], is based on the minimal response dose (MRD), which is the smallest UVA dose that produces a minimal erythema or tanning response. A substantially higher energy dose is required to produce the erythema or tanning response to UVA than is required to produce an erythema or tanning response to UVB, with consequently longer exposure times. The response, evaluated 22–24 h after exposure, is stable, reproducible, and clinically significant in that the action spectra for erythema and tanning [3,4] are similar to those for skin cancer [5] and elastosis in mice [6]. Further, the test is performed on human subjects with skin types I, II, and III, the individuals who have the greatest need for sun protection. The UVA protection factor, PFA, is the ratio of the MRD for sunscreen-protected skin to that for unprotected skin.

5.2.4   Advantages of In Vitro Methods

A major disadvantage of all in vivo methods is that available UV sources, when filtered to remove the UVB portion of the spectrum, do not fully reproduce the UVA portion of the solar spectrum [25].

Sunscreen UVA protection may be evaluated by measuring the product UV transmission spectrum determined in vitro. Once a valid transmission spectrum has been measured for a given product, the degree of UV protection against any effect for which an action spectrum is known may be assessed for any known natural or artificial UV source. The product UV transmission spectrum may be validated by computing the SPF and comparing the SPF determined in vitro to that measured in human subjects. If the SPF calculated from in vitro measurements matches that measured in human subjects, then the UVA protection factor (PFA), or the ratio of UVA protection to overall protection may be computed for any solar spectrum considered relevant to the human exposure situation in question.

5.3   In Vitro Evaluation of Sunscreen Photostability and Critical Wavelength

5.3.1   Photostability

A sunscreen that is photostable has a constant SPF during UV exposure, while a sunscreen that is not photostable (photolabile) has an initial SPF much higher than the labeled SPF, and its SPF diminishes during UV exposure. The SPF measured in human subjects by means of a solar simulator represents the cumulative effective UV dose applied at the time when the cumulative effective UV dose transmitted to the skin reaches one MED. Although a sunscreen with any SPF value can be photostable or photolabile, photostability is desirable because a photostable sunscreen is more likely than a photolabile sunscreen to maintain its labeled SPF value in outdoor sunlight, which generally has a different spectrum from that of a solar simulator. The solar spectrum tends to degrade photolabile sunscreens more effectively than the spectrum of the typical solar simulator. A photostable sunscreen product also requires a lower percentage of active ingredients and thus provides more efficient protection. Perhaps a greater concern is that during the process of photodegradation, photolabile sunscreens may produce free radicals on the skin. The example that follows illustrates in vitro photostability determinations for a hypothetical SPF 30 sunscreen product.

We can model the in vivo behavior of sunscreens on the skin by using an in vitro system, in which the surface of a sunscreen film on a collagen substrate is irradiated and the transmitted UV dose is monitored over time. When the transmitted UV dose in MEDs reaches 1 (1 MED = 20 effective mJ/cm^2), the applied dose is the product SPF. This is analogous to the UV dose at which the MED occurs on human skin. An "ideal" sunscreen has a constant SPF and transmits a constant fraction of the applied dose, while a sunscreen that is photolabile has a diminishing SPF and transmits an increasing fraction of the UV dose. Representative graphs of the applied effective UV dose vs the transmitted effective UV dose for ideal and photolabile ("unstable") sunscreens are shown in Figure 4.

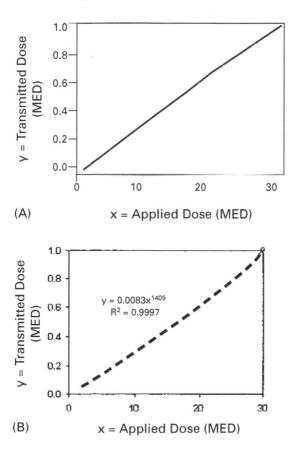

FIGURE 4 Transmitted and applied UV doses for (A) "ideal" and (B) "unstable" (photolabile) sunscreen products rated SPF 30.

For each set of x and y values in Figure 4, we may compute a power curve fit equation of the form

$$y = ax^\beta \tag{9.3}$$

Based on measurements of a large number of products, we have arbitrarily defined a sunscreen with a β value of less than 1.1 as photostable [26].

The UV source is a Solar Light Company Model 16S solar simulator, equipped with a WG320 UVC-blocking filter, a UG-11 filter that blocks visible and infrared light, and a dichroic mirror. Approximately 90% of the effective radiation is in the UVB range.

We measure spectral irradiance from 290 to 400 nm, at 1 nm intervals, using an Optronic Laboratories Model OL754 spectroradiometer equipped with a 6 in. integrating sphere. First we measure the spectral irradiance of the lamp and the spectral irradiance transmitted by a collagen substrate alone, which are both assumed constant. Then we measure the spectral irradiance transmitted by the substrate with sunscreen, at one-minute intervals.

To obtain effective UV doses, we multiply the spectral irradiance value at each wavelength for the lamp by the appropriate erythemal effectiveness factor (see Fig. 2 above) [4] and integrate over wavelength and time. Effective doses are expressed in MEDs.

Next, we apply a thin film of the sunscreen formula (approximately 1 mg/cm^2 before evaporation) to the substrate and allow it to dry for at least 15 min.

Finally, we irradiate the sunscreen film and measure the effective spectral irradiance transmitted through the sunscreen film and substrate, from 290 to 400 nm, at one-minute intervals. Sunscreen photostability is evaluated by calculating the cumulative effective UV dose in MEDs transmitted by the sunscreen product vs the cumulative effective UV dose applied to the surface of the film, until the transmitted dose reaches one MED.

The value of β is obtained from the power curve fit equation, and the estimated product SPF is calculated as the applied UV dose in MEDs for which the transmitted UV dose reaches 1 MED.

5.3.2 Critical Wavelength

The critical wavelength λ_c, proposed by Diffey et al., is calculated by determining the wavelength at which the integral of the thin-film absorbance curve reaches 90% of the integral from 290 to 400 nm [27]. The "ideal" sunscreen would absorb all UV wavelengths equally and would have a critical wavelength of 389 nm. The critical wavelength is a measure of the extent to which a sunscreen product is "ideal" in this respect. A sunscreen with a critical wavelength of 370 nm or higher is considered to be a "broad-spectrum" product [27], although that claim is not permitted under the current Sunscreen Monograph (see later, Sec. 6).

Figure 5 gives the critical wavelengths for the sunscreen products shown in

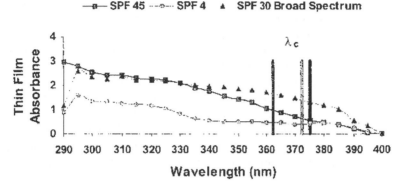

FIGURE 5 Sunscreen absorbance spectra and critical wavelength.

Figure 3. Critical wavelengths are 362, 372 and 375 nm, for the SPF 45, SPF 4, and SPF 30 broad-spectrum sunscreen products, respectively. These curve illustrate that a product with a critical wavelength too short to be considered "broad spectrum" (viz. <370 nm) can still have a high SPF, that a low SPF product can have a critical wavelength above 370 nm and be considered "broad spectrum," and that a photostable product containing Avobenzone generally has a critical wavelength above 370 nm.

6 THE REGULATORY STATUS OF SUNSCREENS

In 1978 the U.S. FDA issued a proposed rule to establish conditions for the safety, effectiveness and labeling of over-the-counter (OTC) sunscreen drug products [10]. The proposed rule, known as the Sunscreen Monograph, was based on the recommendations of the Advisory Review Panel on Over-the-Counter (OTC) Topical Analgesic, Antirheumatic, Otic, Burn, and Sunburn Prevention and Treatment Products. The panel recognized that many products associated with suntanning and sun protection had been tradionally considered to be cosmetics, in accordance with the statutory definition of a cosmetic as "articles intended to be rubbed, poured, sprinkled, or sprayed on, introduced into, or otherwise applied to the human body or any part thereof for cleansing, beautifying, promoting attractiveness, or altering the appearance. . . ." However the panel decided that products intended to be used for prevention of sunburn or any similar condition should be regarded as drugs. Under the Federal Food, Drug and Cosmetic Act [28], drugs are defined as "articles (other than food) intended to affect the structure or any function of the body of man or any other animals. . . ."

Although the Sunscreen Monograph was not a final regulation, FDA has stated that unless a product is the subject of an approved New Drug Application

(NDA), marketing a sunscreen with a formulation or labeling that is not in accordance with an Advance Notice of Proposed Rulemaking (ANPR) or Proposed Rule could result in regulatory action [29].

FDA published the Tentative Final Monograph (TFM) on sunscreens in 1993 [30]. The TFM introduced new labeling and more tedious testing procedures that provoked considerable discussion with the sunscreen industry. In 1997 FDA published an enforcement policy allowing OTC sunscreen products containing up to 3% Avobenzone (Parsol 1789) alone and 2–3% in combination with specified sunscreen active ingredients [31]. In 1998 FDA published a proposed amendment to the TFM to establish conditions for use of products with zinc oxide up to 25% alone and 2–25% in combination with any category I sunscreen active ingredient except Avobenzone [32].

The following feedback meetings have been held by FDA since publication of the TFM [33]:

- June 3, 1998: discussion of sunscreen product formulation
- January 27, 1999: discussion of UVA protection testing methodology
- July 22, 1999: discussion of testing and labeling of sunscreen products with SPF values above 30
- October 26, 1999: discussion of testing methodology for OTC sunscreen drug products with high SPF values

On May 21, 1999, the FDA published the Final Sunscreen Monograph [9]. The Final Monograph covers Part 310, New Drugs; Part 352, Active Ingredients, Labeling, and Testing Procedures; Part 700, Cosmetics Containing Sunscreen Ingredients; and Part 740, Cosmetic Product Warning Statements.

On June 8, 2000, the FDA published an extension of the effective date of the Final Sunscreen Monograph to December 31, 2002 [34], and on December 31, 2001, the FDA published a stay of Part 352. The announcement of the stay stated that the agency "anticipated" that the new effective date of a final rule on Part 352 will not be before January 1, 2005 and that the stay did not affect Parts 310 and 700. The announcement also stated that the agency will be addressing formulation, labeling, and testing requirements for UVA protection and UVB protection [35].

The Final Monograph added paragraphs to 21 CFR 310 stating that any OTC drug product that is not in compliance with the regulation and is introduced into interstate commerce is subject to regulatory action. Part 700 provides that the use of a sunscreen in a cosmetic product for reasons other than sun protection (e.g., to protect product color) must be explained in labeling. Part 740 provides that a suntanning preparation that does not contain a sunscreen must display a warning that the product does not protect users against sunburn. The latter provisions are final regulations.

Thus there is no final regulation for sunscreen formulation, labeling, and testing requirements for UVA protection and UVB protection [35]. As pointed out, however, FDA maintains the position that marketing a sunscreen with a formulation or labeling that has not been approved through the NDA process and is not in accordance with an ANPR or Proposed Rule could result in regulatory action [29]. This appears to make the current Final Monograph sunscreen formulation, labeling, and testing requirements for UVB protection mandatory.

Since the Final Monograph does not address UVA testing and labeling, this area is subject to the provisions of the TFM. At present the only permissible UVA labeling is a statement to the effect that the product offers UVA/UVB protection if its formula contains one or more active ingredients having an absorption spectrum extending to 360 nm or above in the UVA range. Avobenzone, titanium dioxide, and zinc oxide are included in this classification.

7 COSMETICS CONTAINING SUNSCREEN INGREDIENTS

A product can be both a cosmetic and a drug. Examples of "cosmetic-drugs" include deodorants with antiperspirant claims, toothpastes with anticaries claims, antidandruff shampoos, and makeup preparations with sunscreen protection. Cosmetic-drugs must comply with both cosmetic and drug labeling requirements. Section 502(e) of the Food, Drug and Cosmetic Act requires that drug products list all active ingredients on the label. If a product is both a drug and a cosmetic, the inactive ingredients must be listed in accordance with Section 701.3 of the FDA regulations, with some exceptions [33]. Briefly, this means that the sunscreen active ingredients must be listed separately using their drug designations and the other ingredients must be listed in decreasing order by their percent w/w using their International Nomenclature Cosmetic Ingredient (INCI) designations [36].

Perhaps the most common cosmetics containing sunscreen ingredients are moisturizers. Several companies sell "day" formulas containing moisturizers such as petrolatum, glycerine, cyclomethicone, and/or lactic acid, along with sunscreen ingredients such as octyl methoxycinnamate (Octinoxate), octyl salicylate (Octisalate), and titanium dioxide. The "night" formula would contain essentially the same moisturizing ingredients without the sunscreen ingredients. The labeled SPF for such products is usually 15, although some products have labeled SPFs as high as 30. The SPF is almost always a "static" SPF value, rather than "water resistant" or "very water resistant."

Another category is the sunscreen–skin protectant combination. These products are subject to two FDA monographs, the Sunscreen Monograph [9] and the Skin Protectants Monograph [37]. This combination has enjoyed popularity for many years, primarily in lip balms containing sunscreens [36].

Recently a number of products have appeared with "antiwrinkle," "skin brightening," and "skin renewal" claims. These products typically contain vitamins A, C, and/or E, often listed as "antioxidants," or retinol, α-hydroxy acids, or coenzyme Q10. Sunscreen ingredients are typically octyl methoxycinnamate (Octinoxate), oxybenzone, octyl salicylate (Octisalate), and increasingly, Avobenzone. The presence of Avobenzone permits the "contains UVA/UVB protection" claim.

Critical issues for the foregoing products include potential interactions between sunscreen ingredients and the ingredients on which the primary claims are based. Suncreens have been known to reduce the efficacy of moisturizers, and moisturizing ingredients could disrupt the protective film of a sunscreen product. Antioxidants have long been known to exert a protective effect on sunscreen ingredients, enhancing their photostability. These issues present challenges and opportunities in the formulation of innovative multifunctional products.

REFERENCES

1. LI Grossweiner. Photophysics. In: KC Smith, ed. The Science of Photobiology. New York: Plenum Press, 1989, pp 1–45.
2. COLIPA Sun Protection Factor Test Method. Brussels: European Cosmetic, Toiletry, and Perfumery Association, October 1994.
3. J Parrish, K Jaenicke, R Anderson. Erythema and melanogenesis action spectra of normal human skin. Photochem Photobiol 1982;36:187–191.
4. A McKinlay, B Diffey. A reference spectrum for ultraviolet induced erythema in human skin. CIE J 6:17–22 (1987).
5. F de Gruijl, P Forbes. UV-induced skin cancer in a hairless mouse model. BioEssays 1995;17:651–660.
6. L Kligman, R Sayre. An action spectrum for ultraviolet induced elastosis in hairless mice: Quantification of elastosis by image analysis. Photochem Photobiol 1991;53: 237–242.
7. ML Kripke. Immunological unresponsiveness induced by ultraviolet radiation. Immunol Rev 1984;90:87–107.
8. D Moyal. Improved immune protection in humans by a sunscreen with enhanced UVA protection. American Academy of Dermatology, 60th Annual Meeting, New Orleans, February 22–27, 2002 (poster).
9. U.S. Food and Drug Administration. Sunscreen Drug Products for Over-the-Counter Human Use; Final Monograph; 21 CRF Parts 310, 352, 700, and 740. Fed Regis 64(98); May 21, 1999:27666–27693.
10. U.S. Food and Drug Administration. Sunscreen Drug Products for Over-the-Counter Human Use; Advance Notice of Proposed Rulemaking; Fed Regist 43(166); August 25, 1978:38206–38269.
11. Cosmetic, Toiletry and Fragrance Association. CTFA Labeling Manual: A Guide to Cosmetic and OTC Drug Labeling and Advertising, 7th ed. Washington, DC: CFTA, 2001, p 147.
12. NA Shaath. Evolution of modern sunscreen chemicals. In: NJ Lowe, NA Shaath, MA Pathak, ed., Sunscreens: Development, Evaluation and Regulatory Aspects, 2 ed. New York: Marcel Dekker, 1997, pp 3–33.
13. CD Vaughan, SM Porter, JA Gilbert, ML Posten. The South Beach Sunscreen Survey 2001. Cosmet Toiletries 2002;117:55–67.

14. RD Ley. Dose response for ultraviolet radiation A–induced focal melanocytic hyper-plasia and nonmelanoma skin tumors in *Monodelphis domestica.* Photochem Photobiol. 2001;73(1):20–23.
15. ES Robinson, RH Hill Jr, ML Kripke, RB Setlow. The *Monodelphis* melanoma model: Initial report on large ultraviolet A exposures of suckling young. Photochem Photobiol. 2000;71(6):743–746.
16. MF Naylor, BA Smith, DW Smith, et al. High sun protection factor (SPF) sunscreen in the suppression of active neoplasia. Arch Dermatol 1995;131:170–175.
17. SC Thompson, D Jolley, R Mark. Reduction of solar keratoses by regular sunscreen use. N Engl J Med 1993;329:1147–1151.
18. H Schaefer, D Moyal, A Fourtanier. Recent advances in sun protection. In: A Rougier, H Schoeter, eds. Protection of the Skin Against Ultraviolet Radiations. Paris: John Libbey Eurotext, 1998, pp 119–129.
19. RM Sayre, N Kollias, RD Ley, AH Baqer. Changing the risk spectrum of injury and the performance of sunscreen products throughout the day. Photodermatol Photoimmunol Photomed 1994;10(4):148–153.
20. K Kaidbey, and A Barnes. Determination of UVA protection factors by means of immediate pigment darkening in normal skin. J Am Acad Dermatol 1991;25: 262–266.
21. C Irwin, A Barnes, D Veres, K Kaidbey. An ultraviolet radiation action spectrum for immediate pigment darkening. Photochem Photobiol 1993;57:504–507.
22. T Fitzpatrick. The validity and practicality of sun-reactive skin types I through IV. Arch Dermatol 1988;124:869–871.
23. A Chardon, D Moyal, C Hourseau. Persistent pigment darkening as a method for the UVA protection assessment of sunscreens. In: A Rougier, H. Schaefer, eds. Protection of the Skin Against Ultraviolet Radiations. Paris: John Libbey Eurotext, 1998, pp 131–136.
24. C Cole, R Van Fossen. Measurement of sunscreen UVA protection: An unsensitized human model. J Am Acad Dermatol 1992;26:178–184.
25. RM Sayre, PP Agin. A method for determination of UVA protection for normal skin. J Am Acad Dermatol 1990;23;429–440.
26. J Stanfield. Photostability and UVA protection. J Cosmet Sci 2001;52(6):412–413.
27. BL Diffey, PR Tanner, PJ Matts, JF Nash. In vitro assessment of the broad-spectrum ultraviolet protection of sunscreen products. J Am Acad Dermatol 2000;43(6):1024–1035.
28. Federal Food, Drug and Cosmetic Act, 21 U. S. Code 301 et seq.
29. EG Murphy. Regulatory aspects of sunscreens in the United States. In: NJ Lowe, NA Shaath, eds. Sunscreens: development, evaluation and regulatory aspects, 1st ed. New York: Marcel Dekker, 1990, pp 127–136.
30. U.S. Food and Drug Administration. Sunscreen Drug Products for Over-the-Counter Human Use; Tentative Final Monograph. 21 CRF Parts 352, 700, and 740. Fed Regist 58(90); May 12, 1993:28194–28302.
31. U.S. Food and Drug Administration. Sunscreen Drug Products for Over-the-Counter Human Use; Marketing Status of Products Containing Avobenzone; Enforcement Policy, 21 CFR Part 352. Fed Regist 62(83); April 30, 1997:23350–23356.
32. U.S. Food and Drug Administration. Sunscreen Drug Products for Over-the-Counter

Human Use; Amendment to the Tentative Final Monograph; Enforcement Policy, 21 CFR Part 352. Fed Regist 63(204); October 22, 1998:56584–56589.

33. Cosmetics Torletry, and Fragrance Association. CTFA Labeling Manual, A Guide to Cosmetic and OTC Drug Labeling and Advertising, 7th ed Washington, DC: CFTA, 2001, pp 151–152.

34. U.S. Food and Drug Administration. Sunscreen Drug Products for Over-the-Counter Human Use; Final Monograph; Extension of Effective Date; Reopening of Administrative Record, 21 CRF Parts 310, 352, and 700. Fed Regist 65(111); June 8, 2000: 36319–36324.

35. U.S. Food and Drug Administration. Sunscreen Drug Products for Over-the-Counter Human Use; Final Monograph; Partial Stay; Final Rule, 21 CRF Part 352. Fed Regist 66(250); December 31, 2001:67485–67487.

36. K Klein. Sunscreen combination products—Sense or nonsense? J Cosmet Sci 2001; 52(6):408–409.

37. U.S. Food and Drug Administration. Skin Protectant Drugs for Over-the-Counter Human Use; Tentative Final Monograph, 21 CRF Part 347. Fed Regist 48(32); February 15, 1983:6820–6833.

10

Approaches for Adding Antibacterial Properties to Cosmetic Products

Jeffrey Easley, Wilma Gorman, and Monika Mendoza
Stepan Company, Northfield, Illinois, U.S.A.

BACKGROUND

As trends toward multifunctionality have continued, consumer product companies have sought to differentiate their products by expanding the ingredient base of their product lines. The addition of antibacterial agents to a variety of cosmetic products has had a profound impact on the nature of these product line expansions. However, the addition of antibacterial "properties" to cosmetic formulations requires serious consideration. This chapter elucidates the use of some well-known antibacterial agents such as Triclosan, Triclocarban, and PCMX (chloroxylenol) in various cosmetic applications. More specifically, this chapter provides some basic knowledge and practical suggestions for adding antibacterial properties to multifunctional cosmetic products.

1 INTRODUCTION

As stated in the preface to this book, the concept of multifunctional cosmetics has gained prominence over the past several years. The term "multifunctional" can be defined from different perspectives. From a manufacturer's perspective, multifunctional products are those products that can be used to manufacture more than one type of end-use product (e.g., one blend can be used to make a shampoo, a hand soap, and a bubble bath). From a consumer's perspective, multifunctionality more commonly refers to a product's ability to provide more than one major function (e.g., two-in-one shampoos and conditioners). The "multifunctional" antibacterial cosmetics product market consists of such products as liquid hand soaps, body washes, and even lotions. But despite the ongoing use of these products, there is still some controversy centering on their application in finished cosmetic products.

The marketing of products containing antibacterial agents has come under heavy scrutiny. The antibacterial "fad," as many call it, is viewed as a potential threat by some who say that continued use of such products could ultimately promote the growth of resistant strains of microorganisms. The generation of these new strains could conceivably expose us to new diseases. Some who disagree with this school of thought, however, argue that antibacterial agents like Triclosan have been used in homes and in hospital environments for more than 30 years with no apparent "side effects." Those with this opposing view suggest that research has not established a link between antibacterial products and bacterial resistance. So with all these issues, why is there still a market for antibacterial cosmetic products? Why add antibacterial functionality to multifunctional cosmetic products?

If we stop to think for a moment from the customers' perspective, some interesting "theories" arise concerning the continuing trend to add antibacterial properties to multifunctional cosmetics. Could it be that consumers view products of these types as being value-added with respect to "the war on germs"? This is certainly a possibility. The addition of antibacterial agents to cosmetic products may give consumers that added bit of confidence that they have rid themselves of all dangerous microorganisms. Plain soaps (those without antibacterial agents) are just used for cleaning—not for the removal of dangerous microorganisms. This thought process might also exist among consumers.

On the other hand, consumers (especially the aging segment) are on a health kick. They are on a rather successful quest to lead long, active, productive lives. They have control over their diet, their activities, and to some degree their genetics. They wear sunscreens, reduce stress levels, and buckle up. What is left? The next war front to guarantee optimal health is controlling their external environment. One way to achieve this is to reduce the infectious bacteria that cause colds, diseases, and maladies (many of which children bring home with them from day care, schools, and play groups). Thus the war on bacteria and the antibacterial explosion is permeating every conceivable cleaning product and household item, including cutting blocks, shower curtains, and toys. Before long, the phrase "Cleanliness is next to godliness" will be replaced by "Germ-free is the only way to be!"

In this chapter, we discuss some experiential approaches to the art and science of adding antibacterial functionality to cosmetic products. Major topical areas include commonly used antibacterial agents, the incorporation of antibacterial agents in surfactant systems, testing for the presence of antibacterial agents, microbiological testing, stability and shelf life, and future trends related to the use of antibacterial agents in cosmetics. The information presented in this chapter provides some practical insights on how to successfully incorporate antibacterial agents into multifunctional cosmetic products.

2 SO WHAT IS AN ANTIBACTERIAL AGENT?

Very simply stated, an antibacterial ingredient is an active ingredient used to kill or control the growth of bacteria. The term is often used interchangeably with "antimicrobial." The mode of action for killing or inhibiting the growth of bacteria varies with the type of antibacterial agent used. Triclosan, for example, is thought to block the active site of an enzyme needed by many bacteria and fungi for survival. The blockage of this active site in essence prevents bacteria from making fatty acids, which are necessary for various aspects of cell construction. Quaternary compounds also work by destroying the cell wall of bacteria.

Figure 1 presents the chemical structures of some commonly used antibacterial agents.

3 CONSUMER FEAR OF GERMS

Historically, consumers have relied on cleanliness to reduce bacterial contamination. We wash to remove as many pathogens as possible. With food poisonings, viruses, and the common cold, health care concerns on are the rise. This germ phobia has resulted in an outburst of antibacterial products: soaps, lotions, facial cleansers, cutting board products, dishwashing soaps, kitchen and bathroom cleaners, countertops, kitchen appliances, pillows, sheets, mattress pads, kitty litter, children's toys, socks, athletic shoes, toothbrushes, sponges, and even toothpaste. Many people have an irrational fear of germs, and they are demanding better and safer products. The market is responding with a wide range of antibacterial products. Parents want to protect their children from the dangers of bacteria. Let us not forget the growing contingent of baby boomers and the "Gen Xers," pursuing their quest for health and fitness. With more travel, day care, and public transportation, today's consumer is determined to fight the war on germs.

The antibacterial soap market is a 1 billion-dollar-a-year business. Between 1992 and 1998, 673 antibacterial products were introduced on the market according to a report in the *Seattle Times* [1].

Yet one might still ask, Why add an antibacterial agent? Depending on their active ingredients and specific formulation, antibacterial soaps or washes are effective against the bacteria that cause odor, skin infections, food poisoning,

Antibacterial Agent	Chemical Structure
Triclosan 2,4,4'-trichloro-2'-hydroxydiphenyl ether	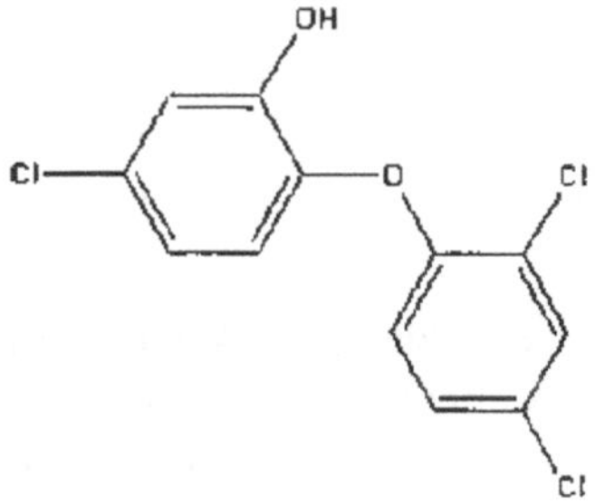
Trichlocarban 3-(4-chlorophenyl)-1-(3,4-dichlorphenyl) urea	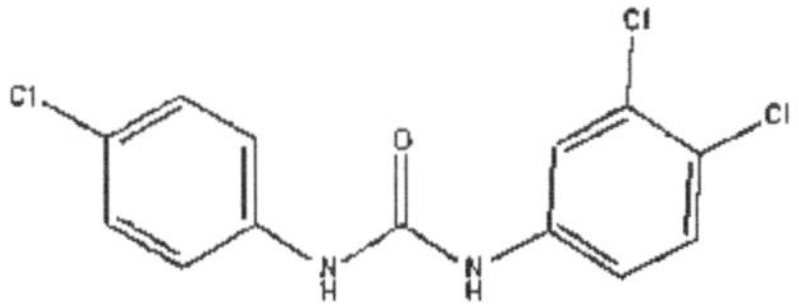
Quaternary Ammonium Compounds n-Alkyl Dimethyl Benzyl Ammonium Chloride	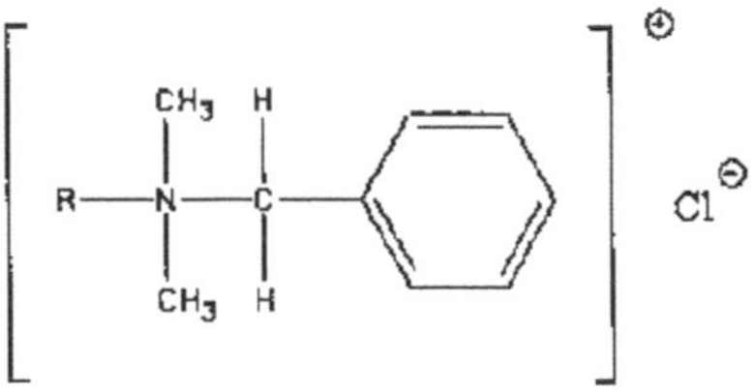

FIGURE 1   Structures of some antibacterial agents.

intestinal illnesses, and other commonly transmitted diseases (the common cold). Triclosan, the most commonly used antibacterial agent, adds staying power to soap by killing germs and stopping bacteria growth for as long as 6 hours.

Antibacterial wash products have been used safely by consumers for over 30 years. In fact, antibacterial soaps were first introduced in the 1920s to control odor-causing bacteria. They are regulated by the U.S. Food and Drug Administration (FDA).

Why this sudden boom in antibacterial products? We have a better educated, more aware public. Hand washing is recognized by the Centers for Disease Control and Prevention as one of the most important means of preventing germs from spreading. Washing your hands removes harmful bacterial such as staphylococci, streptococci, *E. coli,* and salmonella. These bacteria can cause illnesses such as skin infections, strep throat, and food poisoning. However, regular soaps do not kill the germs. They do loosen germs from the skin and increase water's ability to wash them down the drain. Antibacterial soaps remove 97% bacteria on hands, while regular soaps remove about 70%. The FDA claims that washing hands with an antibacterial soap results in reduced bacterial growth on the skin compared with washing with plain soap, since a very small amount of the antibacterial agent remains on the skin after rinsing and provides continued control of the growth of bacteria. Personal cleansing and household cleaning products that contain an active antibacterial or antimicrobial ingredient provide extra protection against germs, including those that may cause disease. These agents kill or control the growth of microorgansims and help prevent germs from spreading.

Liquid antibacterial handsoaps are the most popular, widely used, and best accepted product in the market today. It is well known that germs are most often spread by hands through person-to-person contact. The common cold is solely responsible for an estimated annual loss of 60 million days of school and 50 million days of work. Second to a cold, some 5.5 million visits to doctor's offices each year are due to skin infections. To every movement there is a flip side, and it is necessary to state that there is some concern about the everyday need for antibacterial products. Antibacterial products do offer protection over soap if you have an open cut or sore that could become infected. They certainly have a place in hospitals, restaurants, and child care centers, where the level of sanitation must be at its highest.

As mentioned earlier, the FDA is concerned that the overuse of antibacterial products could lead to new strains of resistant bacteria. However, some bacteria are actually helpful. These bacteria are necessary to fight other bacteria and some prepare us for more virulent strains by building up our resistance. Antibacterial bar soap products were introduced in 1970 with brand names like Irish Spring and Life Buoy. In 1972 Dial bar soap was introduced, but it did not make an anti bacterial claim until the 1990's. Lever 2000 antibacterial deodorant soap contains Triclosan. PPG's Safeguard antibacterial deodorant soap, advertised as an all-family germ fighter, contains 1.2% trichlorocarbanilide (Triclocarban).

3.1 Liquid Hand Soaps

The first liquid soaps were solutions of soaps used in public washroom dispensers. Liquid soaps entered the mass market and appeared in consumer bathrooms in 1979 when Minnetonka launched Softsoap, quickly followed by products from Dial and Andrew Jergens. These products enjoyed an attractive growth to about the mid-1980s and captured 8–9% of the soap market. In 1986 Liquid Dial with antibacterial properties was introduced. By 1990–1991 antibacterial liquid soaps sales grew 20%. In 1993 they had captured 14% of the soap market in dollar terms. By 1996 these products plateaued. But the interest did not. Manufacturers focused on product niches and succeeded in launching in a third boom! The consumers are educated and ready for the next wave to hit. So add two-in-one products such as dishwash liquid/antibacterial handsoap or an antibacterial with lemon juice (Kitchen Softsoap).

It is not always possible to wash with soap and water as needed. Instant hand sanitizers provide an effective alternative that is easy to use. This convenient product was originally designed to supplement employee hand washing in the health care and hospitality industries. Alcohol-based instant hand sanitizers kill 99.99% of disease-causing germs within 15–30 seconds (product claims vary) without water. In 1998 Gojo Industries, regarded as the originator of this category, introduced its Purell line of instant hand sanitizers, quickly followed by Dial, Colgate-Palmolive Softsoap, Unilever's Helene Curtis Suave, Del Laboratories' Sally Hansen, and Avon Products.

For the trendy consumer, the message is "Good hygiene is cool!" In upscale markets, you can find designer antibacterial products from Tommy Hilfiger, Banana Republic, and Limited Too; Instant Shimmer Antibacterial Hand Gel from Bath and Body Works has silvery glitter.

For the very young consumer there are fun and effective antibacterial products in bright colors, tempting sweet smells, and brands such as Kiss my Face enticing children to practice better hygiene. Kids use the scented soap that contains 0.33% Triclosan by weight, and parents can determine by smell whether hands have been disinfected. Products contain natural ingredients such as aloe vera and glycerin that are gentle to children's hands. Further excitement is added by making cleanup fun by licensing children's toy brands and television characters such as Minnetonka Brands's Sesame Street and Loony Toons antibacterial hand gels. Convenience is the appeal for disposable hand towlettes. Johnson's antibacterial towlette is alcohol free, contains benzalkonium chloride, and is billed as a "gentle bacterial solution to help you clean away dirt and reduce bacteria."

For the aspiring chef, Amway Body Series offers an antibacterial liquid hand soap that cleans skin and neutralizes food odors like those of onions, garlic, and fish. Dermatologist tested and allergy tested, the product is concentrated, and only half the usual amount is claimed to destroy 90% of surface bacteria.

3.2 Body Washes

The trend did not stop with hand washing. The obvious expansion was in body wash. Although popular in Europe for many years, in the United States liquid body wash products were originally considered a luxury pampering gift item saved for Christmas, birthdays, and Mothers Day. Body wash products gradually showed up in the mainstream consumer stores. The acceptance of antibacterial handsoaps resulted in the development of several antibacterial body washes. Dial Plus antibacterial (1994), Dial Plus Ultra skin antibacterial (1995), and Soft Soap gentle antibacterial (1996) are examples. Dial's antibacterial moisturizing body wash is two-in-one antibacterial product (containing moisturizers) that provide antibacterial protection with Triclosan, a trusted antibacterial agent.

3.3 Antibacterial Lotions

Antibacterial lotion was a new segment in the hand and body lotion categories. As with the antibacterial liquid soaps, this too was first used in health care and food service. In 1996, BMS Keri antibacterial hand lotion was introduced, followed by Lever Vaseline Brand Intensive Care antibacterial hand lotion with germ protection. There is no evidence that using antibacterial lotions reduces the incidence of any disease.

3.4 Active Ingredient

The active ingredient in most antibacterial products is Triclosan, an agent that damages the cell walls of bacteria, slowing their ability to multiply. The FDA has concluded that Triclosan is safe for use in consumer products. Gel (no-rinse) products contain ethyl and/or isopropyl alcohol. Chloroxylenol (PCMX) is the active ingredient in Sunshine's antibacterial soap, and the claims are as follows: exhibits broad-spectrum antimicrobial action, effective against gram-positive and gram-negative organisms, as well as yeast and fungi including MRSA (methicillin-resistant *Staphlococcus aureus*).

3.5 Other Antibacterial Cosmetic Products

3.5.1 Acne Products and Antiseptic Cuticle Treatments

Avon ClearSkin medicated antibacterial foaming face cleanser contains 0.3% Triclosan. J&J's Clean and Clear contains Triclosan and kills problem-causing bacteria without overdrying. Cuticura medicated antibacterial bar contains 1% Triclocarban and advertises that it "cleans and controls oil and germs that can cause blemishes." Sally Hansen's antiseptic cuticle treatment kills germs on contact, fights infection, and soothes painful torn cuticles. The product is designed to kill germs that can lead to infection in torn, damaged cuticles. It contains 0.13% benzalkonium chloride.

Avon Foot Works is a therapeutic cream for the relief of cracked heels. Containing 0.13% benzalkonium chloride and 4% lidocaine, it provides first aid to help guard against skin infection in minor cuts, scrapes, and burns.

3.5.2 Toothpaste

The FDA approved Colgate Total, the first toothpaste containing an antibacterial agent (0.3% Triclosan) and the first dentifrice clinically proven to help fight gum disease (gingivitis) in adults (the clinical study did not involve children). Colgate conducted studies that showed that Total (in combination with chloride) reduced plaque by 11.9% in the first trial and 9.3% in the second. This equates to a reduction in gum disease by 19.3 and 29.0%, respectively. It is not fully understood how Triclosan works in your mouth. Triclosan is considered to be a drug, and all new toothpastes containing it must be approved by the FDA.

3.5.3 Antibacterial Toothbrush

Antibacterial toothbrushes, made from a plastic called Microban, are also available. Microban has been found to inhibit the growth of bacteria. The toothbrush is part of the Reach line of toothbrushes manufactured by Personal Products Company. The toothbrush's antibacterial ingredient is said to inhibit "the growth of bacteria that may affect the plastic in the handle." The EPA oversees use of Triclosan in plastic products. Antibacterial toys also are made of plastic that contain Triclosan.

4 INCORPORATING ANTIBACTERIAL AGENTS INTO SURFACTANT SYSTEMS

Incorporating antibacterial agents into surfactant systems is often a formidable task, even for the experienced formulator. The choice of antibacterial agent, the amount of agent used, the types of surfactants used, and processing conditions all impact the effectiveness of the formulation effort.

In choosing an antibacterial agent, several factors should be kept in mind:

Cost of the antibacterial agent
Proposed efficacy claims (different agents inhibit or destroy different microorganisms: e.g., gram-negative or gram-positive organisms)
Product availability
Compatibility with formulation ingredients (includes such components as surfactants, solvents, dyes, fragrances, and other promotional additives)
cGMP (current good manufacturing procedures) requirements, if applicable

Intent to make a ready-to-use product or a concentrate

Intent that antibacterial ingredient be added by the manufacturer or by the user

Regulatory requirements (e.g., guidelines proposed by the FDA's tentative final monograph, where applicable)

Compatibility with potential by-products

Safety and risk factors associated with the handling of the antibacterial agent

Stability and environmental fate of the antibacterial agent

This list is not exhaustive, but it does provide some of the key factors associated with choosing an antibacterial agent. Once these and any other pertinent factors have been reviewed, we can proceed to investigate the proper amounts to be used in a given system. The planning process described is not necessarily a linear one. Several "stages" of the planning process often overlap and/or occur simultaneously. As mentioned previously, Triclosan, Trichlocarban, PCMX, and alcohols are commonly used as antibacterial agents. Quaternary ammonium compounds have also been successfully used as antibacterial agents.

The amount of antibacterial agent to use depends not only on the type of antibacterial agent, but also on the proposed product application. For example, Triclosan is considered to be a "broad-spectrum" antimicrobial agent. In other words, it is capable of being effective against a variety of bacteria, molds, and yeasts. For deodorant soap bars or spray deodorants, 0.15–0.30% by weight of Triclosan has been shown to be effective. Surfactant-based hand disinfectants typically incorporate anywhere from 0.40% to 2.0% by weight of Triclosan, but 1% is preferred. Alcohol-based surgical scrubs typically require 0.20–0.50% of Triclosan (with 0.30% being the preferred amount). Different surfactant systems along with a variety of other components may necessitate deviation from recommended levels to achieve required efficacy. Keep in mind that recommended use levels are just that—recommended. If product claims are to be made, it is ultimately the manufacturer's responsibility to be sure that a product is efficacious. Methods for quantitatively evaluating the level of agent in a finished product are very briefly discussed in the next section. Some basic microbiological tests are also mentioned.

Chloroxylenol is also a commonly used antibacterial agent. In some formulations, it has been used effectively at approximately a 3% by weight level. Once again, you must evaluate the use of PCMX in your formulation. It may take more or less to develop an efficacious product. The same basic guidelines apply to the use of Trichlocarban, alcohols (such as isopropanol or ethanol), and quaternary ammonium compounds. Do not assume that recommended levels are appropriate. Always have your product tested for efficacy if claims are to be substantiated.

A variety of surfactants and other ingredients are used to formulate multi-functional cosmetic products. Surfactant types often include (but are not limited to) α-olefin sulfonates, alkanolamides, betaines, ether sulfates, alkyl sulfates, and amine oxides. Other components may include such items as chelating agents, conditioning agents, film-forming agents, and of course water. Tables 1–3 presents some "starter" formulations as examples.

The hand soap and body wash formulations shown in Tables 1 and 2 contain Triclosan as the antibacterial ingredient, while the premium hand soap formulation (Table 3) contains a quaternary ammonium chloride as the antibacterial agent. All of these products are considered to be multifunctional because they not only perform their stated functions (as hand soaps and body wash), but they also provide an extra level of protection against germs by inclusion of the antibacterial agents.

In many cases, it is important to follow any mixing instructions as directed. Not doing so could cause instability problems with your formulation. Pay close attention to the recommended procedures for incorporating the antibacterial agent into your product(s). The manufacturer of the antibacterial ingredient typically provides the necessary mixing instructions.

Another factor that may impact the efficacy of your product is pH. Be sure to consult the appropriate literature from the manufacturer of your antibacterial agent for specifics.

A word on antibacterials versus preservatives. A preservative or preservative system is used for the purposes of protecting your product from decay, discoloration, and/or spoilage. Antibacterial agents are specifically designed to either reduce or to eliminate microorganisms. So even though some antibacterial agents are capable of usurping some of the functionality of a preservative, it is still wise in most cases to employ a separate, effective preservation system in your product(s).

You should also be aware that antibacterial agents such as Triclosan, PCMX, and Trichlocarban are considered to be over-the-counter (OTC) drugs, and as such, they are regulated by the U.S. Food and Drug Administration (FDA). Because of the OTC Drug designation of these products, it is strongly advisable that "current good manufacturing practices" be put into place before embarking on the manufacture of your product. It is beyond the scope of this chapter to discuss the details of setting up a cGMP program. In some instances, you may need to solicit the services of an outside consultant. Suffice it to say that establishing a cGMP program entails such matters as keeping accurate records of all analyses and product batches. In addition, manufacturing plants that make antibacterial products must be registered with the FDA; and warehousing and distribution procedures must be written, monitored, and signed off appropriately. There are several other requirements, as well. If you are unfamiliar with cGMP, locate a company with experience in this area and try to set up a visit. It will be time well spent.

TABLE 1 Starter Antibacterial Hand Soap Formulation with Triclosan[a]

Ingredients	Amount (% by weight)	Functionality	Mixing instructions
Deionized water	As needed to make 100	Solvent, carrier	1. Charge vessel of appropriate size with deionized (DI) water.
BIO-TERGE® S-HS[b]	25.00	Surfactant blend	2. Start agitation.
Polyquaternium-7	0.50	Film-forming agent	3. In a separate vessel, pre dissolve the Triclosan in the surfactant blend under mild heating (50–60°C).
Aloe vera gel	0.05	Biological additive	4. Add the surfactant–Triclosan mixture to the DI water and continue to mix.
Disodium EDTA	0.10	Chelating agent	5. Add the polyquaternium-7, aloe vera gel, disodium EDTA, and hydrolyzed silk protein.
Hydrolyzed silk protein	0.40	Biological additive	6. Mix until homogeneous.
Triclosan	0.30	Antibacterial agent	7. Adjust to desired pH with citric acid or sodium hydroxide.
Dye, fragrance	As needed		8. Cool the batch to an appropriate temperature, then add fragrance, dye, and preservative.
Preservative	As needed		

[a]This formulation is a typical antibacterial hand soap that has excellent flash foaming characteristics.
[b]BIO-TERGE® S-HS contains sodium C14–C16 olefin sulfonate, lauramide DEA, and cocamidopropyl betaine. BIO-TERGE is a registered trademark of Stepan Company.

TABLE 2 Starter Antibacterial Body Wash Formulation with Triclosan[a]

Ingredients	Amount (% by weight)	Functionality	Mixing instructions
DI water	As needed to make 100	Solvent, carrier	1. Charge vessel of appropriate size with DI water.
STEPANOL® A-HS[b]	30.00	Surfactant blend	2. Start agitation.
Glycerin[c]	2.00	Humectant	3. In a separate vessel, pre dissolve the Triclosan in the surfactant blend under mild heating (50–60°C).
Polyquaternium-7	0.50	Film-forming agent	4. Add the surfactant/Triclosan mixture to the DI water and continue to mix.
Disodium EDTA	0.10	Chelating agent	5. Add glycerin, polyquaternium-7, and disodium EDTA.
Triclosan	0.30	Antibacterial agent	6. Mix until homogeneous.
Dye, fragrance	As needed		7. Adjust to desired pH with citric acid or sodium hydroxide.
Preservative	As needed		8. Cool the batch to an appropriate temperature, then add fragrance, dye, and preservative.

[a]This formulation is a water-white, low-odor, mild body wash with excellent foaming and viscosity-building characteristics. This product is excellent for sensitive skin and for incorporation of delicate fragrances.
[b]STEPANOL® A-HS contains sodium laureth sulfate and cocamidopropyl betaine.
[c]U.S. Pharmacopeia grade.

TABLE 3 Starting Formulation for Premium Antibacterial Hand Soap Based on Quaternary Ammonium Compounds[a]

Ingredients[b]	Amount (% by weight)	Functionality	Mixing instructions
BIO-SOFT® N1-7 (alcohol ethoxylate)	1.70	Soil removal	Add first eight ingredients to water and mix well. Heat to 60–70°C and continue mixing for 30 minutes or until all material is dissolved. While mixing, cool to room temperature and adjust pH to 5.5–6.5 with citric acid. Add fragrance, dye, and preservative. No salt is necessary for viscosity adjustment.
AMPHOSOL® CA (cocamidopropyl betaine)	16.67	Primary surfactant	
AMMONYX® CDO special (cocamidopropylamine oxide)	7.81	Secondary surfactant	
AMMONYX® CO (cetamine oxide)	3.33	Conditioning	
NINOL® LMP (lauramide monoethanolamine)	2.00	Foam stabilizer	
STEPAN® PEG 6000 DS (PEG-150 distearate)	1.00.	Thickening agent	
BTC® 835 (n-alkyldimethyl-benzyl-ammonium chloride)	2.00	Antibacterial agent	
Disodium EDTA	0.20	Chelating agent	
Citric acid (50%)	As needed	pH control	
Fragrance, dye, preservative	As needed		
DI water	As needed to make 100	Solvent, carrier	

[a]Quaternary-based antibacterial hand soap (ABHS) formulations offer a unique alternative to traditional antibacterial liquid soaps. This starting formulation provides broad-spectrum antibacterial coverage, good viscosity, foaming, and mildness. In addition, the formulation is clear, nearly colorless, and imparts a pleasant feel to the skin.
[b]BIO-SOFT®, AMPHOSOL®, AMMONYX®, NINOL®, STEPAN®, and BTC® are all registered trademarks of Stepan Company.

5   TESTING FOR THE PRESENCE OF ANTIBACTERIAL AGENTS

When you are developing a multifunctional product with antibacterial agents, it is beneficial to determine the presence of the antibacterial agent incorporated and quantitate its amount. The FDA requires manufacturers to determine the amount of a regulated substance in a product when using a controlled substance such as an antibacterial agent (Triclosan, e.g., is considered to be an over-the-counter drug).

Various methods can be used to analyze for the presence and amount of antibacterial agent in your multifunctional product. Most test methods can be obtained directly from the company supplying the antibacterial agent. Typically, the industry uses gas chromatography to test for agents like PCMX, Triclosan, Triclocarban, and alcohols. The test method for gas chromatography calls for the sample to be dissolved in a solvent (when needed) and injected into the gas chromatograph to obtain a peak area for the antibacterial agent. Then it is compared quantitatively against a standard of the antibacterial agent's solutions using an external standard calibration curve based on peak areas. Quantitation is achieved by either a three-point calibration curve or by a single-point external standard technique [1].

The level of quaternary ammonium compounds (quats) is determined by titration with standardized sodium lauryl sulfate (SLS) solution. Two types of titration are available: potentiometric titrations and two-phase titrations. A preferred potentiometric titration involves an aqueous solution of quat that is adjusted to pH 10.5 and titrated potentiometrically with standardized SLS by means of a nitrate ion selective electrode. The titration leads to the formation of a water-insoluble complex between the quaternary compound and the SLS. The end point is determined by the electrode's response to the increasing concentration of SLS. A two-phase titration with SLS, with bromophenol blue as a visual indicator, is used by laboratories that do not have potentiometric titration equipment. The end point is reached when the first purple color appears in the aqueous top layer [2].

Testing for the presence and quantities of the antimicrobial agent is necessary when the multifunctional product containing the antibacterial agent is undergoing micro-efficacy testing. The FDA advises manufacturers on the types of test and the results that are needed to make specific claims. The guidelines for tests and kill results are outlined in the FDA's Tentative Final Monograph (TFM).

The type of claim(s) you want to make on your product and the type or category of product you have will determine the type of microtesting needed. For instance, there are products that are applied and then rinsed off, like hand soaps and body washes. To make an "antibacterial handwash" claim, you may need to perform in vitro and in vivo tests that include minimum inhibitory concentration (MIC), time-kill, general use handwash methods, and residual efficacy tests (e.g., Agar Patch) [3].

Furthermore, there are products that are applied and left on, like lotions, sanitizers, and deodorants. Several years ago the FDA advised manufacturers to simply follow the TFM with modifications appropriate to leave-on products. This works for the hand sanitizer type of product, but extensive changes need to be made in the TFM methods for products that rely upon long-term antimicrobial action (i.e., lotions).

The FDA supplies monographs for most product types out on the market. Yet some products, like toothpaste and toothbrushes, do not fit into any of the categories mentioned thus far. The information needed for testing parameters may be obtained directly from the FDA. Also, the FDA has a very informational website (http://www.fda.gov).

Antibacterial agents are also found in products that do not make any claims except for cosmetic and deodorizing claims. Therefore, these products do not have to follow the TFM, nor are they obliged to undergo rigorous testing. For instance, deodorants usually contain an antibacterial agent to help control odor by killing the odor-causing bacteria. However, because only a deodorizing claim is stated on the product, time, money, and energy are not spent on achieving compliance with TFM regulations.

6 SUMMARY AND FUTURE TRENDS FOR ADDING ANTIBACTERIAL FUNCTIONALITY TO COSMETIC PRODUCTS

It appears that multifunctionality is here to stay. And adding antibacterial agents to your cosmetic products is one way of achieving this goal. There are a variety of antibacterial agents that can be used. Triclosan, PCMX (chloroxylenol), Trichlocarban, alcohols, and quaternary ammonium compounds are all examples. These types differ with respect to their effectiveness against different types of organisms. There are a wide variety of antibacterial, multifunctional products on the market. Many of these products are targeted for specific cohorts. There is controversy with respect to the use of antibacterial agents. One camp thinks that continued use of these products will help to create new strains of bacteria for which we would have no resistance. Others point out that agents such as Triclosan have been used for more than 30 years with no signs of new bacterial strains developing. But despite all these rumblings, antibacterial agents continue to be used in cosmetic products.

When considering the addition of antibacterial agents to a product, you should address questions such as How much should I use? and How do I effectively incorporate the agent? And since antibacterial products are considered to be OTC drugs, cGMP guidelines should be established and put into place. Quantitative methods for assaying antibacterial agents should be available, as well as a means to microbiologically verify the efficacy of your finished formulations.

Two recent products appearing in the marketplace are water-white and sensitive-skin formulations. The trend for clear, light color formulations has resulted in an increased use of alkyl ether sulfate (AES) versus α-olefin sulfonates (AOS). Further product segmentation and "appeal-ability" to a wide range of consumers—infants, babies, toddlers, children, preteens, teens, young adults, and seniors—will yield creative packaging and fragrances.

REFERENCES

1. C Micheels, "Germ Resistance: Beyond the Hard Surface," *Seattle Times,* August 1999, p. 31.
2. GC Short Form Method for Irgasan 300. Ciba-Geigy Customer Service Department.
3. ASTM D12.12 Subcommittee, Standard Test Method for Disinfectant Quaternary Ammonium Salts by Potentiometric Titration, D 5806-95. 1996 Annual Book of Standards. Vol 15.04. Philadelphia: American Society for Testing and Materials, 1996, pp 612–615.
4. Topical Antimicrobial Drug Products for Over-the-Counter Human Use; Tentative Final Monograph for Health-Care Antiseptic Drug Products. 59(116) Fed Regis 31402–31452 (June 17, 1994).

11

Claims Support Strategies for Multifunctional Products

Lawrence A. Rheins
DermTech International, San Diego, California, U.S.A.

1 INTRODUCTION

The 1990s provided the global personal care industry with a multitude of multifunctional cosmetic products for hair, skin, nails, and other areas. This trend will continue certainly into the first decade of the new millennium and beyond. Therefore, this chapter was written to aid cosmetic chemists in successfully developing testing programs for multiclaim substantiation. It is important for cosmetic chemists to have an awareness of these specialized claim support techniques because the increasingly vigilant marketplace [i.e., Federal Trade Commission (FTC), National Advertising Division of the Better Business Bureau (NAD), Food and Drug Administration (FDA)] will no doubt "gently" direct manufacturers to develop claims that are scientifically based and defensible, along with a strong profile of safety data prior to market launch. Following a review of the current tenets of safety testing, specific examples of claims substantiation for multifunctional personal and skin care products are described. The chapter concludes by describing what approaches (such as molecular biology) may be used for developing novel product efficacy support in the future.

2 SKIN CARE

Safety testing of skin care products is an important prerequisite to successful market launch for two-in-one, three-in-one, and all-in-one products. This is because the skin, as the largest organ of the body, is an extraordinarily complex and dynamic organ. To maintain normal homeostasis with the internal and external mileu of the body, the stratum corneum along with the major epidermal cell types [i.e., keratinocytes, melanocytes ("pigment cells"), Langerhans cells (the immune macrophage of skin), Merkel cells (resevoir for skin neural peptides), and T-lymphocytes, plus a myriad of cutaneous cytokines] determine whether perturbation to the skin and/or its appendages during application of cosmetic skin care products results in the potential development of either irritant or allergic contact dermatitis. Furthermore, one needs to evaluate the more common dermatosensorial safety issues (e.g., itching, burning, tingling, stinging phenomena) that may lead to barriers for ultimate marketing success of complex performance designed personal care products [1–4].

Our recommended approach involves following a tiered safety program. As validated alternatives to animal testing continue to remain a technical and regulatory hurdle for skin safety, other in vitro approaches have successfully emerged [5]. In our laboratory we typically begin by evaluating novel active ingredients and/or finished formulations by using healthy, viable, surgically excised human skin tissue obtained from routine cosmetic or plastic surgical procedures or discarded porcine skin from a local meat processing plant. In this manner one literally has the entire biology of the skin present for conducting routine skin safety procedures. The test articles are applied to the whole viable skin explants under semioccluded exposure conditions.

After 4 hours of exposure, punch biopsies (3 mm) are performed at the treated and control sites. The biopsy specimens are histologically fixed and stained with a variety of vital stains including stains for skin lipid integrity and inflammatory infiltrate. Simple light microscopy (240×) can provide an abundance of information regarding initial skin safety with objective precise histopathological evaluation. This quick, accurate skin safety screen can then provide the product development oxicology team with specific information on which test articles to place into the traditional industry standard predictive patch tests. This particular laboratory utilizes the cost-effective 14-day cumulative irritation study plus a challenge patch application to assess initially cumulative irritation "mildness" and sensitization (i.e., "allergy") potential in one clinical study. Infrequent adverse reactions that have occurred with multifunctional personal care products also led this particular laboratory to recommend 4–6 weeks of in-use studies as an absolute key to ensuring safety prior to a market launch of complex personal/skin care–type products.

For example, the complex interactions of an α-hydroxy acid (AHA)/sunscreen and botanical excipient product are quickly complicated with routine consumer use of the consumers additional over-the-counter (OTC) or prescription dermatological and even systemic medications. The "polypharmacy" culture of the United States has presented an additional safety concern for understanding and approximating near- and long-term safety in the use of multifunctional cosmetic products.

Briefly, during the 4- to 6-week study to determine safety in use, subtle skin condition symptoms (e.g., itching, burning, stinging, tingling) and even more significant irritant or allergic reactions can be evaluated under real-world consumer use conditions. Furthermore, one must remember that millions of end users with common yet compromised skin conditions (sensitive skin, atopy, psoriasis, chronic eczema, etc.) will also want to purchase and routinely use these complex products. This rather sizable niche population of consumers with compromised skin usually is excluded from routine skin, hair, and nail safety studies, yet the relatively long 6-week in-use study can provide the manufacturer with safety information for this important population as well. The completion of the foregoing safety tests provides the manufacturer and raw material distributors of these multifunctional personal care products with a compelling and comprehensive safety database for market entrée.

3 CLAIMS SUBSTANTIATION FOR MULTIFUNCTIONAL SKIN CARE PRODUCTS

The perceived and/or real performance characteristics for multifunctional skin care products requires a clinical trial design that can objectively quantify multiple clinical end points that are supportive of each specific marketing claim. During the last few years this laboratory has conducted several studies with products containing glycolic acids (AHAs), as well as skin-lightening active ingredients (e.g., hydroquinone, botanical tyrosine inhibitors).

3.1 Fine Lines and Wrinkles

Claims for one product evaluated by our staff included "reduces the appearance of fine-line wrinkles" and "lightens darkness around the eyes." A clinical study design for this type of claims support required (1) identifying a statistically significant number of test subjects based on the derived biological end points for the particular claim, (i.e., the more quantatively precise the biological data, the fewer test subjects required), (2) use of clinical end points that have appeared in the peer-reviewed scientific literature, and (3) detection limits of the desirable clinical end point that provides precision and reliability, which in turn can demonstrate statistical differences as small as 15% between competitive products.

For the measurement of "fine-line wrinkles reduction appearance," a combination of clinical 35 mm close-up photography coupled with silicon replicas analysis provides demonstrable quantitative changes in perioral or periocular fine-line wrinkles. The image analysis scanning of the silicon replica provides a level of quantitative precision that can help differentiate performance of one product versus another in a statistically significant fashion ($P < 0.05$).

3.2   Skin Lightening

To evaluate the skin-lightening effect of a product, we perform punch biopsies (2 mm) in the periauricular area of the ear at baseline prior to treatment and following 8 weeks of topical treatment to the contralateral ear region. Following 8 weeks, a second 2 mm punch biopsy sample is obtained from the treated periauricular region of the ear. The skin biopsy specimens are snapped, frozen, and stained with, for example, S-100 monoclonal antibody (which stains specifically for pigment cell and melanin presence when an indirect immunoperoxidase staining procedure is used). Figure 1 shows untreated skin (baseline). One can see dendritic melanocytes at the basal region of the epidermis (arrows). Figure 2 shows S-100 staining following 8 weeks of topical treatment. Note the subtle yet quantitative reduction in the absolute number of visible pigment-producing melanocytes. Although this difference is not clinically significant to the test subject, *t* is an objective quantitative observation of the product's true performance. A bioinstrumental, immuno-histochemical approach coupled with 35 mm clinical photography provides a very comprehensive set of multifunctional marketing claims for this particular two-in-one skin care product.

3.3   An Example of Combination Claims

Another interesting multifunctional skin care product includes a three-in-one product containing san protection factor (SPF) a moisturizer, and skin-lightening performance characteristics. Manufacturers of moisturizing products in general tend to focus on consumer use of moisturizers in regions that are cold and low in humidity. Although dry skin in these climatic regions does indeed present with the usual flakiness, itching, and general consumer discomfort, consumers in regions with hot weather and low humidity present with some different cosmetic skin care needs.

These consumer concerns not only consist of the standard dry flakiness, but the cosmetic aesthetic issue of photodamage, including unwanted darkening pigmented regions of the skin. When one evaluates habits and practices, these particular consumers typically wear clothing allowing exposure to ultraviolet (UV) light of the legs and arms approximately 10 months of the year.

Thus, a three-in-one product that conditions and lightens the skin and offers UV protection would typically require a study design to encompass a multitude of biological end points for claims substantiation. First, one would need to perform

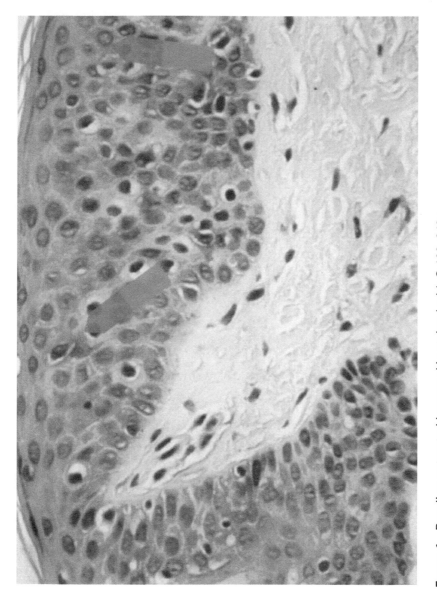

FIGURE 1   Baseline untreated human skin stained with S-100, 240×.

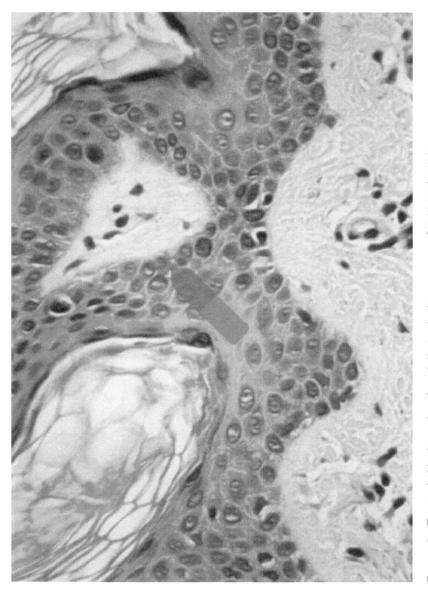

FIGURE 2   Treated skin 8 weeks after daily topical treatments S-100 stain 240×.

a standard static SPF-15 sunscreen study complying with the most recent guidelines of the FDA monograph [6].

The second component of the claims would require a standard 14-day dry skin regression study [7]. This approach usually involves a 7-day washout period, 2 weeks of topical treatment with dedicated clinical skin evaluation, and finally a regression period to determine how long it takes for skin moisturization effects (i.e., duration) to return to baseline levels. This well-established industry approach involves clinical assessment of the skin, the degree of skin flakiness based on a standardized scale of 1 to 4, and bioinstrumental assessment that objectively quantifies changes in moisture loss by means of transepidermal water loss (TEWL), changes in resistance/capacitance, or magnetic resonance imaging. The nuclear magnetic resonance (NMR) approach, albeit somewhat new to the skin care industry, can evaluate water loss in the skin in an extraordinarily precise and quantitative fashion and offers a high level of reproducibility.

The third claim of skin lightening for this type of three-in-one product would entail at least two approaches. First, areas of heavily pigmented UV-damaged skin would need to be well demarcated for repeated sequential clinical 35 mm photography from a standardized camera system such as the industry-validated Canfield System. Ultraviolet light pigmentation on the legs is often complicated with various telangiectasia, purpura, and simple spider veins, thereby necessitating a standardized camera system photographing a templated area for evaluation of lightening skin care products.

In addition to the standardized clinical photography, one would use a ChromaMeter to provide additional information on subtle yet quantitative changes (i.e., changes not perceivable to the human eye, yet providing a numerical score to augment the clinical photography data set). Again the combination of clinical, bioinstrumental, and 35 mm photography provides an excellent claims substantiation tried for this unique three-in-one skin care product.

3.4 Nail Care

In a different study we evaluated a two-in-one nail care product that was crafted to offer claims of "improvement in the appearance of the cuticle (flakiness, redness), and conditions the fingernail to help prevent nail splitting, rough edges" of the nail. This particular study involved designing a clinical protocol utilizing again 35 mm close-up photography and histological immunofluorescent staining observations of fingernail biopsy samples. In this study product design, women with long fingernails, and "damaged" cuticles were impaneled. Baseline photography of the cuticles on day zero (no treatment) and fingernail clipping biopsies (day 1 of treatment) were performed. Prior to application, the nail care products received 15 µg of fluoroscein isothiocyanate (FITC) fluorescent dye. The nail product was applied three times a day for 5 days of treatment. Comparison of the photographs for day zero (Fig. 3) and for day 5 of treatment (Fig. 4) demonstrates improvement in cuticle appearance (less redness, flakiness, rough edges) versus baseline (day zero). Furthermore, Fig. 5, revealed little penetration into the nail plate following one day of treatment with the dye treated nail product (arrows) yet, by day 5 one can see a demonstrable amount of nail product penetrating into the nail plate, (Fig. 6). One can easily measure differences under the light microscope with an ocular grid, between the topical nail treatments of days 1 and 5. Again, a combination of clinical close-up 35 mm photography along with immunohistological staining of the fingernail biopsy samples provided multiple claims support for this very interesting two-in-one nail care product.

3.5 Hair Care

3.5.1 Safety Issues

One extracutaneous appendage that continues to receive high marketing and product development interests is hair, and the multifunctional hair care products are much studied. The safety concerns discussed earlier certainly apply to hair care products; however, the focus is not as intense because in general (reactive products such as colors and perms are an exception), hair care products are not intended to react with biological substrates. Therefore, this section focuses on claims support, not safety evaluations. Likewise, the chapter does not focus on new hair growth, since products capable of inducing it are truly pharmacologic drugs and require regulated testing, but instead explores how one might evaluate hair care products with respect to "color tone" and ingredient penetration.

3.5.2 Claims Support Strategies

Color Tone. Our laboratory has studied hair color steadfastness by utilizing hair tresses and analytical chemistry. Briefly, hair tresses are treated with hair dye according to the manufacturer's guidelines. Then over the course of 5 days of treatment, the tresses are gently shampooed with various water conditions, taking into account water hardness, temperature, and so on, at 10 minute intervals.

Aliquots of the washings are then subjected to standard spectrophotometric scanning to evaluate changes in baseline and in treated color hair tone. This approach can also be used when one is comparing current products with market innovators to perform simple pilot screening studies in developing claims for parity or superiority. The data generated from these pilot studies can then in turn be used to develop definitive clinical studies for ultimate marketing claims.

Penetration Studies. Further, to evaluate ingredient penetration into the hair shaft or even deeper into the hair unit (cuticle), hair tresses again can become

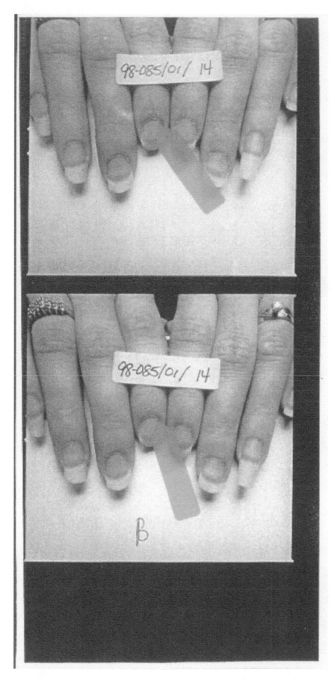

FIGURE 3   Baseline clinical evaluation of damaged nail and cuticles.

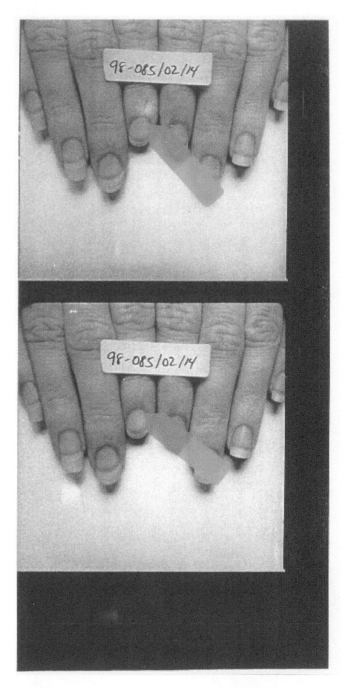

FIGURE 4 Cuticle and nails following 5 days of topical treatment.

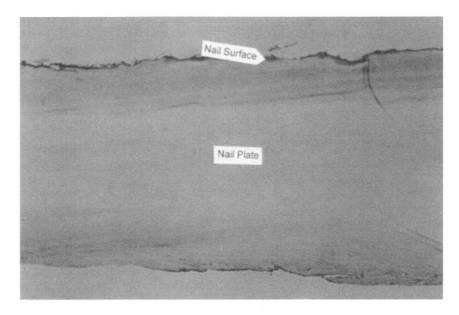

Figure 5 Fingernail biopsy at day 1 of topical treatment, Baseline 250×.

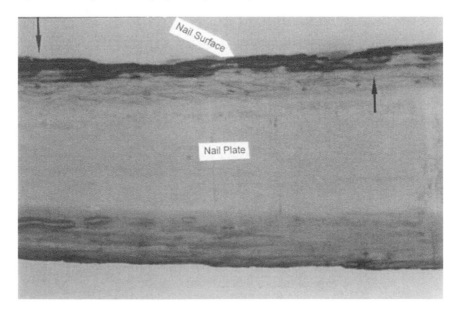

FIGURE 6 Fingernail biopsy at day 5 of topical treatment with refined jojoba oil, 250×. Note the penetration of the product into the nail plate as apposed to the nail at day 1 of treatment.

a valuable testing tool. One can simply radiolabel the hair care preparation with something such as tritiated thymidine or carbon-14. Tritium is a low beta emitter, and with relatively simple radiation safety precautions one can generate some eloquent autoradiograph clearly demonstrating the penetration of various chemical entities into the hair shaft and deeper for "hair nutrient claims." Again, one can perform the testing over a 5-day time period for 10 minutes per treatment to establish the kinetics for ingredient penetration [8].

For those studies, where working with radioactive isotopes is simply not an option, one can look to specific fluorescein probes, coupled with fluorescent epimicroscopy, to track ingredient penetration. Although such techniques clearly are not as quantitative and precise as the radiolabeled approach, one can generate some compelling data in comparison to appropriate controls. One of the downsides of this experimental approach is that fluorescein can nonspecifically stain keratin molecules, thereby producing at times a significant amount of nonspecific "noise." However, with some simple trial-and-error sequences using various concentration and ratios of product to the fluorescein dye, one can derive some very striking photography claims [9].

If one uses double labeling such as fluorescein isothiocyanate (green) and phycoerythrin (red) in testing one hair care product against another, one could conduct a clinical study again taking hair samples every day over the course of 5 days of treatment. Typically one would use a regimen of hair products with a cleansing shampoo, conditioner, and even a hairstyling product. However, by using double-labeling fluorescent microscopy techniques, it becomes possible to confirm that the penetration observed is indeed due to penetration of the product ingredient into the hair shaft, not an artifact of fluorescein chemistry. From a marketing perspective, moreover, these fluorescent probes can indeed provide a high-impact, visually compelling color photography for a variety of multifunctional hair care products.

There are many other requirements for claims support related to multifunctional products including deposition of active ingredients, hair strength, and elasticity. These are commonly used in the industry and are discussed elsewhere.

4 FUTURE APPROACHES

It is clear to this author that the increasing use of functionally active raw ingredients in multifunctional personal care products will continually require innovative claims testing approaches to accurately quantify claims in a compelling, defensible fashion to meet the needs of the market place (as defined by FTC, NAD, FDA, etc.) as well as the end users' ultimate needs.

The completion of the human genome project may indeed open the door for even more sophisticated claims substantiation for multiregimen skin and personal care products. One could clearly envision individually design (custom-based products that are quickly formulated based on an individual's own genetic makeup and, particularly, and users' skin types). What just 5 years ago would have seemed like science fiction is today clearly becoming identifiable science fact.

Our laboratory developed a technology called DermPatch that can noninvasively recover messenger ribonucleic acid (mRNA) from the skin [10]. Recall that the mRNA encodes for the various proteins in the skin—collagen, fibrin, elastin, cytokine, to mention only a few. Furthermore, this technology recovers proteins in femtomole amounts, essentially a one- or two-molecule detection level capability [11].

This technology is able to quantify molecular events occurring at the surface of the skin following topical application of multifunctional skin/personal care products. As such, one can envision having the ability to finally address true "mechanism of action" of various cosmetic products, thereby providing the product formulator the tools to make changes to specific functional or cosmetic product attributes based on the molecular protein translation of events of interest. These molecular events are occurring constitutively as part of the normal homeostatic physiological functioning of skin, nail, and hair. What is exciting is the ability to rapidly and objectively measure a variety of either stratum corneum or epidermal events to the skin, nail, or hair appendages at a molecular level following routine use of cosmetic products. Currently our laboratory is using this technology for differentiating irritant versus allergic skin reactions [10]. Additional studies are under way to use this technology for measuring in vivo antioxidant anti-inflammatory attributes of natural botanical-based products.

In summary, the global arena of multifunctional personal care products, synthetic and natural, as well as combinations thereof, will continue to evolve well into the first decade of the new millennium to meet various consumer needs. Technology-designed products based on peer-reviewed scientific literature provides at least one solid approach to developing even more compelling claims for marketing multifunctional personal and skin care products. The key will always remain that the active ingredients of formulated products must indeed be safe as required by industry-accepted, practiced safety studies. Although the claims may reveal product performance differences in the skin, nail, or hair when some of the methods noted in this chapter are used, these biologically measurable events are infinetesimally small, hence should portend no potential health significance to the consumer.

Our ability to objectively quantify a biological event in the skin, nails, or hair following perturbation with the cosmetic product does not necessarily imply drug effects provided the claims are written and structured to convey only an aesthetic consumer-perceivable effect, not a drug effect. As an industry, we need to embrace the new millennium and explore new identifiable claims testing methodologies that will ultimately propel this industry into the next level of performance, thereby meeting and exceeding future consumer needs.

REFERENCES

1. Nordlund JJ, Abdel-Malek AZ, Boissy RE, Rheins LA. Historical review of pigment cell biology. J Invest Dermatol 89:535, 1989.
2. Nordlund JJ, Amornsiripanitch S, Rheins LA, Abdel-Malek ZA, Boissy RD, Bell M. The role of melanocytes in epidermal inflammatory/immune responses. Pigment Cell Res 1:101, 1988.
3. Rheins LA, Noravec RA, Nordlund ML, Trinkle LS, Nordlund JJ. The role of antioxidants in skin immune reactions: The use of flow cytometry to determine alterations in Ia positive epidermal cell in allergic contact dermatitis. J Soc Cos Chem 40:101, 1989.
4. Rheins LA. What's new in cutaneous toxicity? J Toxicol—Cutan Ocul Toxicol 11:225, 1992.
5. DeWever B, Rheins LA. In Vitro Toxicology: Skin2™—An in vitro human skin analog. HI Maibach, ed. Larchmont, NY: Mary Ann Leibert Press, 1994, p 121.
6. U.S. Food and Drug Administration. United States Sunscreen Final Monograph (SFM), May 1999.
7. J Wang S, Kislaliough, Brener M. The effect of rheological properties of experimental moisturizing creams/lotions on their efficacy and perceptual attributes. Int J Cosmt Sci 21:167, 1999.
8. Inoue T, Sasaki I, Yamaguchi M, Kizawa K. Elution of SI00A3 from hair fiber: New model for hair damage emphasizing the loss of SI00A3 from cuticle. J Cosmt Sci 51, 2000.
9. Cohen C, Kollias N, Forrest M. Fluorescent photography in the assessment of hyperpigmentation of photodamaged skin. J Invest Dermatol 102:568, 1994.
10. Morhenn VB, Chang EY, Rheins LA. A noninvasive method for quantifying and distinguishing inflammatory skin reactions. J Am Acad Dermatol 41, 1999.
11. Morhenn VB, LA Rheins. A novel method for diagnosing contact dermatitides. Am J Contact Dermatit (submitted).

12

The Role of Packaging in Multifunctional Products

Craig R. Sawicki
TricorBraun, Clarendon Hills, Illinois, U.S.A.

1   INTRODUCTION

Packaging is an important tool in designing multifunctional products. Some products require a unique functional delivery system to be efficacious; others rely on special packaging to convey their multifunctional nature to the consumer. The package design maybe determined by specific product requirements such as the need to keep ingredients separated during storage, to mix ingredients only upon dispensing, or to dispense the contents in a controlled, metered fashion. Some products require some sort of activation by the consumer such as shaking or mixing. Each of these requirements must be considered when one is designing packaging for multifunctional products. This chapter discusses ways in which packaging can support multifunctional products in terms of both functionality and appearance. It also discusses factors to consider in the selection of packaging materials.

2   ACHIEVING MULTIFUNCTIONALITY

2.1   Ingredient Separation

We begin with a discussion of two key ways in which packaging can support multifunctional: by keeping ingredients separated and by allowing special dispensing. The need to keep ingredients separated until delivery may be important for a number of reasons. For example, some products cannot be homogenized for reasons of efficacy; in other products the active ingredients may not be stable when mixed with other ingredients. Some products use one ingredient as a catalyst to activate some performance characteristic. In other cases, ingredients are separated only to give some indication of dual function.

Whatever the reason, there are only a few ways within the packaging options to keep products separate until used. The easiest way is to use separate vessels. This method employs two or more separate bottles, tubes, packets, or dispensers that the consumer will open, mix, and use. A common example of a product using this approach is epoxy glue. This type of product is frequently packaged in separate cans or jars. The consumer opens each container, applies a portion to a mixing area, stirs to activate, and applies. A newer, more evolved dual-delivery system involves a dual-chambered syringe (Fig. 1) that keeps the products separated.

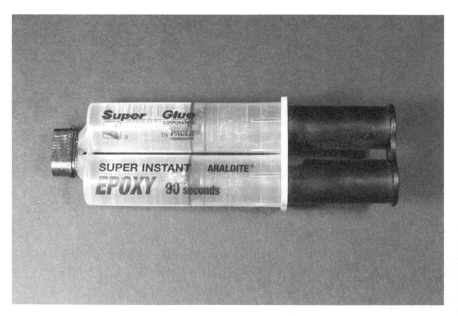

FIGURE 1   Dual-chambered syringe (Courtesy of Superglue Corporation.)

The plunger forces product from each chamber out two individual orifices to a mixing area. The consumer then mixes the components and applies the product. This method also affords a reasonable metering of each of the two components, since the plungers of the syringe are attached to each other.

Another example of dual dispensing is the Unilever Dove Nutrium Mosturizer package (Fig. 2). This package utilizes two separate bottles attached to each other and dispensed through a single large oval flip-top cap with two orifices. The consumer is expected to squeeze out and mix the products in the hand before application. Some advantages as well as limitations exist with this concept. The advantage is that this package enables complete segregation of the ingredients. Since the moisturizer is quite viscous, the designer placed the bottles in an inverted position so that gravity always keeps the product at the orifices. This also allows

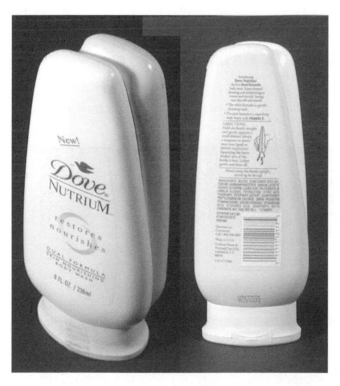

FIGURE 2 Dual dispensing package utilizing two separate bottles attached to each other and dispensed through a single large oval flip-top cap with two orifices. (Courtesy of Unilever Corporation.)

complete evacuation of the product, a definite advantage for the consumer. However, since the largest and most visible area is the side opposite the attaching panels, that would be the preferred area for labeling or decorating. Shelving the product at retail then would hide the second bottle. To compensate for this effect, the package designer chose to offset the alignment of the front bottle slightly from the back, to show both compartments.

Another example of individual vessels is the KMS Hair Reconstructor (Fig. 3). In its most recent form, this product employs two separate D-shaped bottles that are snapped together to form a round.

Separation of ingredients does not always require separate containers. Note for example the Liquid-Plumr package (Fig. 4). This product has two separate ingredients, one of which is a catalyst that causes violent foaming. The container separates the ingredients by means of a wall between the chambers. With certain types of molding (extrusion blow molding in this case), the center wall of molten plastic is pinched within the mold, creating the individual chambers. This method is clearly applicable when squeezing of the package for dispensing is appropriate or when both ingredients are liquid enough to be poured out. Other molding methods available for integral wall separation include injection molding. Some heat-sealed, bottom-filled tubes enable a wall for separation. One example utilizing this process is Enamelon toothpaste (Fig. 5). Much like the Liquid-Plumr package, this tube has a wall through the center separating the ingredients. It too relies on

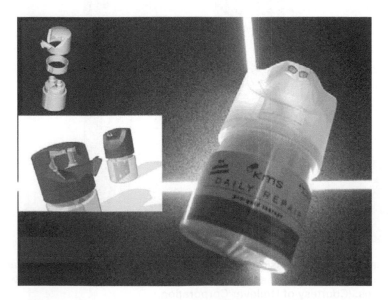

FIGURE 3 Example of individual vessel employing two separate D-shaped bottles snapped together to form a round. (Courtesy of KMS Research, Inc.)

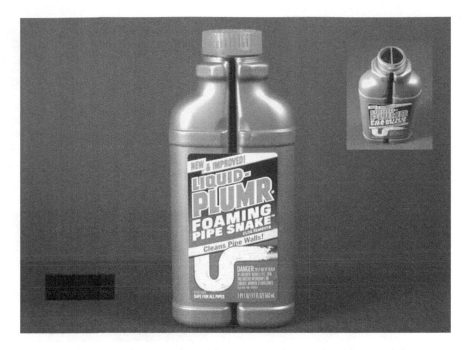

FIGURE 4 The container produced by means of extrusion blow molding, separates the ingredients by means of a wall between the chambers. (Liquid Plumr courtesy of the Clorox Company.)

squeezing to dispense and as such has the potential for a variance in amount dispensed of each ingredient.

2.2 Specialized Metering

Another factor to consider in the design of multifunctional packaging is metered dispensing. To rely on the squeezing of a container to dispense product is inherently inaccurate, especially when the product employs dual ingredients. It would require equal pressure on each container to dispense like amounts. Although exact measure is likely noncritical in such products, this variable creates another difficulty. If the consumer consistently dispenses unequal amounts, one chamber will evacuate faster than the other, leaving the consumer with the perception of wasted product or a single ingredient remaining that is unusable.

In the case of KMS product described in connection with Fig. 3, two separate lotion pumps are used for dispensing. The pump nozzles are directed toward each other with an overcap that also functions as a unified pressure area for the pumps. This not only affords the ability to pump the product uniformly, but also

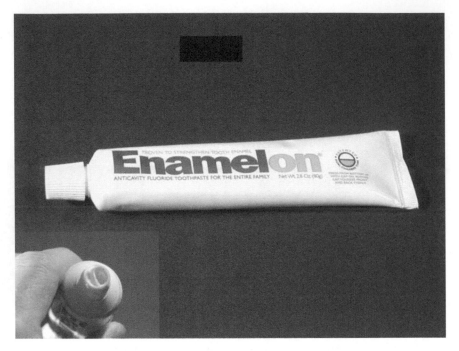

FIGURE 5 Heat-sealed, bottom-filled tube with wall through center, separating ingredients. (Courtesy of Enamelon, Inc.)

allows the pump to be locked during travel. With the pump in the unlocked position, the user simply presses the overcap cap down to pump the two ingredients into the hand for mixing and application. Some new spray products are now utilizing mixing technology. Products that may be appropriate for such a dispenser are those that need a catalyst or even concentrates to be mixed with water upon spraying. Some even provide the ability to vary the dosage of each ingredient depending on product concentration or manufacturer's instruction.

Metering of multifunctional products can also help support a unique marketing position. Note for example the Variosun suncare product and dispenser (Fig. 6). This container utilizes a complex mechanism that allows the consumer to mix a desired suntan lotion with a specific sun protection factor (SPF). The package uses two separate chambers channeled into two separate pumping mechanisms that employ a dial to control the amount of each component dispensed. Again, variance of individual product dispensing causes one chamber to empty before the other. As such, this design enables each side to be refilled with a replacement cartridge that will fit only the proper side of the package.

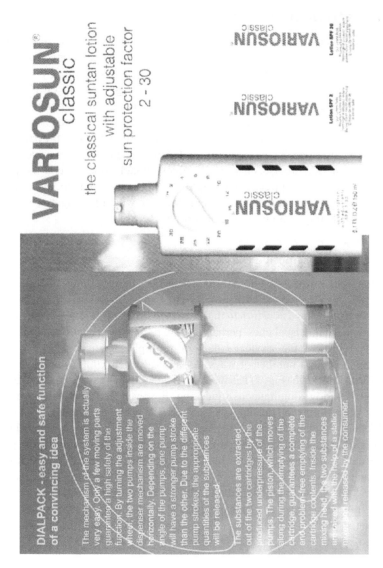

FIGURE 6 Container utilizes a complex mechanism that allows the consumer to mix a desired suntan lotion with a specific sun protection factor (SPF). (Photo courtesy of Variotec.)

3   PACKAGING AS A MARKETING TOOL

In marketers' attempts to differentiate their products from those of competitors, value is added by claiming and delivering a product that performs multiple tasks. That added value needs to be expressed clearly to the consumer by visual representation. According to marketing firms, the average product on a store shelf receives 0.3 second of visibility to an individual shopper. If and only if the shopper's attention is grabbed, the product will gain the full 3 seconds necessary for a purchase decision to be made. Within that small window of time, the package must accurately describe what it does, portray its benefits, and show its value over competing products. Three seconds barely gives enough time to read the product's name and review the price. Obviously everything else needs to be visually self-evident. The next section describes some ways in which packaging can help support the marketing of a multifunctional product.

3.1   Shape: Distinctive Silhouettes

The functional aspects of product delivery may dictate much of the package's shape. Having covered the package's function and how its shape lends itself to the products delivery, we now turn to the visual attributes of its shape. Some products, however, have no visual cues, perhaps owing to delivery function, and the need to visually represent the product's dual or multiple function. This can be done through shape in a number of ways. As noted earlier, Unilever's Dove Nutrium Moisturizer package (Fig. 2) has the advantage of dual chambers to convey its distinction. To allow simultaneous squeezing, however, the two bottles are attached to each other, joined on the flat panels. When the package is shelved in a store, the dual feature might not be noticed unless a consumer picked up or closely inspected the product, thus ascertaining that the bottle in front is only part of the package. Therefore the designer chose to slightly offset the alignment of the back bottle to accentuate the second part. The back bottle was produced in a different color to further contrast the function. Although the separate bottles are a functional necessity in this example, a package's contours can simulate the same image. A simple change to a normal flowing shape can suggest a dual function. Shapes such as a pinched-waist bottle or an hourglass can suggest dual chambers.

3.2   Color

Package color can also relay messages to the consumer. Although subtle, color plays an important part in visual recognition. Colors are more easily associated with certain brands than words or symbols. One can hardly argue the association of the primary color of red with Coca-Cola, or the color yellow with the golden arches of McDonald's. Even further, color has become a common tool used to differentiate the different flavors or choices within product types. Flavors themselves frequently are identifiable by color. Lemon yellow, orange orange, green for lime, and purple for grape are all easily identified. Within the salsa category, it is almost universal that red indicates hot, yellow medium, and green mild. Another example is coffee—red or orange indicates regular coffee and green signals decaffeinated. It is interesting that red has been the brand identifier for both Folger's and Hills Brothers' coffee for decades. However, the classification of regular and decaf was stronger than the need for brand identification. And as such, the decaf flavor of both those brands forced green labeling. Shoppers have come to rely on color for product information and identity.

Multifunctional products frequently combine products that can be identified by color. A recent product introduction is Colgate 2in1, a combination toothpaste and mouthwash (Fig. 7). Mouthwash is most frequently blue or green and toothpaste is most frequently white. The package itself, as well as its labeling, are predominantly blue and white. Even the advertising shows a painter splashing a canvas with white toothpaste and blue mouthwash to create an abstract painting of the product. Deodorants and antiperspirants are almost always identified by the same colors. And as such the packaging conveys that combination in many cases.

Subtlety is rarely a tactic used in marketing. However, a case can be made

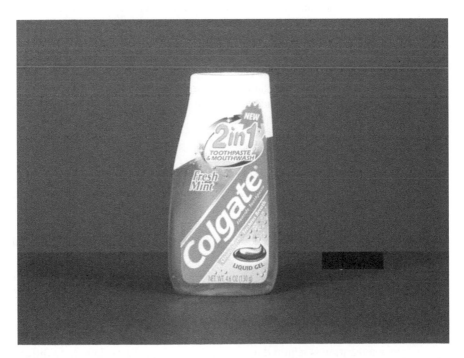

FIGURE 7 Multifunctional 2 in 1 combination product: toothpaste and mouthwash components are identified by color. (Courtesy of Colgate, Inc.)

for the use of complex colors to express duality. Primary colors are exactly that, primary and singular. The primary colors are red, yellow, and blue; all other colors are some combination of those. White is also seen as a noncomplex color, and sometimes black as well. A subtle message (maybe too subtle) of multiplicity is given by using colors such as green, purple, or orange. Pearlescents and translucents also give the impression of complexity. Car manufacturers recently adopted a range of colors that look different in different lighting conditions. This tactic can also be used in packaging.

The most straightforward method in the use of color would be in dual- or multicompartment packages. The individual chambers should be manufactured in separate contrasting colors. If the individual compartments are manufactured as a single unit, then a clear or frosted package should be used with contrasting colors of the product itself. As always, the package should speak for the product and should be as informative and provocative as possible.

3.3 Surface Finishes

As with color, contrasting finishes can also be used to convey multifunctionality. With multicompartment containers, texture on one compartment versus a glossy smooth surface on the other accentuates the contrast. Even on a single-compartment container, selective placement of textured labeling or graphics can indicate the product function. These textures, as with all visual clues, should be as dramatically different as possible. Glass decorating has for some time utilized a method of masking a selected area of a bottle, then spraying with a color or frost. The masked area then retains its original smooth finish. Also used to create that finish is a method for acid etching: the bottle is first masked, then acid is applied by either dipping the bottle or spraying to acquire the desired effect.

3.4 Labeling/Decorating

A picture is worth a thousand words. This phrase has become a cliché because it is so self-evidently true. A multifunctional product's label allows the marketer to use words, pictures, and colors to shout the message, differentiate the product, and grab attention. The label or decorating affords the ability to graphically represent the product and to tell how or why it should be purchased and used. Verbal instructions are frequently more important for products of these types than for conventional products. Especially for products that require mixing of two or more substances, both the method and the reason need to be expressed. The marketer cannot assume that the consumer knows why the substances need to be separated before use. The information should be presented in a way that explains that the product is better because of the separation, that one part acts as a catalyst to the other, or that separation is required to deliver the product. To explain these differences and the label presentation, some examples are necessary.

KMS Research is a California-based manufacturer of professional hair care products. For some years, they had a conditioning product called Hair Reconstructor (Fig. 3). The packaging for the original product was two separate half-ounce packets, much like ketchup packets, that the consumer or stylist would tear open, mix together in the hands, and apply to the hair. It was necessary to express clearly to the consumer that one packet acted as a catalyst to the other, and to retain the product's efficacy, the contents of the two packets needed separation until delivery. This was accomplished by labeling the packets "part A" and "part B" and by printing the top half of "part A" in beige and the bottom half in white, while "part b" was white on the top and beige on the bottom. The advantage that KMS had with this product was the opportunity for the stylist to verbally explain the benefits of the product and its function. Even so, the product had to be able to explain itself to the stylist. The KMS "Reconstructor" product evolved into a unique two-compartment dispenser whose function is explained in Sec. 2.2, the labeling and decoration, however mimicked the packet printing.

A fine example of catalyst separation and the labeling explanation is the two-chamber Liquid-Plumr package (Fig. 4). This "foaming pipe cleaner" product foams upon the mixing of the two ingredients. The label clearly shows the two products pouring as liquids from the bottle and becoming a dense foam flowing through the drain. The label's graphic depiction indicates that one of the ingredients is a foaming catalyst and that the product's components not only need to remain separate until use but that when activated, the product does something that others do not. In short, the label should communicate how the product functions, what it does, why it is multifunctional, and whether the ingredients are separate. A clear graphic is better than words, but a clear description verbally, preferably on the back panels, adds to consumer education.

4 SELECTING PACKAGING MATERIALS

A question commonly asked by product development staff is What packaging material should I use? When packaging materials were few and their differences and attributes obvious, this was an easy question to answer.

No more. Today the answer to the question of packaging material selection is not always clear-cut. For any combination of function, aesthetics, economics, and application, the manufacturer has several materials to choose from.

4.1 Critical Factors in Packaging Selection

The manufacturer must weigh several vital factors to arrive at the best packaging decision the following checklist will help you to keep these important elements in mind.

Barrier requirements as determined by your product ingredients and shelf life

Graphic and aesthetic requirements as determined by your product positioning

Dispensing requirements as determined by your product characteristics and market appeal

Process requirements as determined by available technology and operational control

Strength, weight, and safety requirements as determined by processing, distribution, and end use application of your product

Economic requirements as determined by cost and price factors in your market

Environmental and resource impact

This checklist can help you to choose from among the multitude of plastics, glass, metal, and paper alternatives being offered in today's market.

4.2 Plastic Materials

The "general" category is composed of bottles made from polyolefins, polystyrene, and polycarbonate thermoplastics. Thermoplastic materials can be repeatedly hardened and softened by the respective application of cold and heat.

4.2.1 Polyolefins

Polyolefins have traditionally been the workhorses of the marketplace. Included in this group are all density grades of polyethylene, as well as polypropylene and the ionomers. At this time, because of processing problems and packaging disadvantages, the ionomers are not being commercially sold for blow-molding purposes.

Polyolefin applications in various end markets include hair and skin care products, household cleaners, milk, liquid margarine, and syrups. Polyolefins' versatility is reflected in the massive tonage sold and processed in the world today.

Polyethylene Resins. The basic ingredient from which polyethylene resins are made is ethylene monomer, a gas derived from natural gas or the cracking of crude oil. Ethylene polymers may be made through the use of several processes, which produce commercial materials of varying densities.

ADVANTAGES OF POLYETHYLENE

Low to moderate stiffness for flexibility and good resistance to breakage.

Relative inertness exhibiting outstanding chemical resistance. Only hot solvents such as toluene, xylene, or benzene will dissolve polyethylene.

Good barrier for moisture vapor transmission in higher density grades that allow use with water-soluble products.

Good squeezability, especially in lower density grades. Readily available material that is easy to process.

DISADVANTAGES OF POLYETHYLENE

Relatively high transfer or permeation of taste ingredients
Relatively low hot-fill temperature tolerance
Poor barrier for nonpolar materials or gases
High distortion level with oil-based products
Poor clarity and gloss finish
Brittleness at low temperatures

Polypropylene Resins. The basic ingredient of polypropylene resin is propylene monomer; a normal by-product of catalytic or thermal cracking of gas oil in gasoline production. Propylene requires further purification for polymerization. Propylene polymers are generally made by means of a low-pressure process. Both homo- and copolymer resins are produced. Copolymer grades generally utilize ethylene monomer to improve impact strength.

ADVANTAGES OF POLYPROPYLENE

Lowest density thermoplastic available today; more cubic inches of plastic per pound
Moderate stiffness and relatively good impact properties at room temperature
Good moisture vapor transmission rate
Product contact clarity
Excellent inertness and resistance to chemicals at room temperature
Little tendency to stress cracking
Good capability of hot-fill applications up to 165–185°F
Improved surface finish and slightly higher gloss than polyethylene
Moderately good resistance to distortion by oil products

DISADVANTAGES OF POLYPROPYLENE

Some deterioration of polypropylene's ability to withstand impact at temperatures of 40°F and below
Semiclear in unfilled state
Relatively poor barrier for gases and nonpolar materials
High permeation of taste ingredients
Poor scuff and mar resistance

(When polypropylene is biaxially oriented, these disadvantages are lessened and clarity is markedly improved.)

4.2.2 Polystyrene

With the advent of injection–blow molding, polystyrene has found many uses in packaging, mainly in the medicinal and health areas, where it is used for products like aspirin tablets, capsules, vitamins, and petroleum jelly. Because its offers a relatively poor barrier to gas and moisture, polystyrene's use has been limited to products with a relatively short shelf life.

Polystyrene monomer is made from coal tar and petroleum gas. The initial step is to combine benzene and ethylene to make ethyl benzene, which is then purified and dehydrogenated to produce styrene monomer. General-purpose polystyrene is the simple polymerized form of styrene monomer. All general-purpose polystyrenes are not identical. Considerable variation is possible within the family by changing weights and their distributions. Addition of comonomers such as acrylonitrile and methyl methacrylate increases the versatility of the resins. Major differences are in hardness, rigidity, gloss, structural properties, solvent resistance, and impact.

ADVANTAGES OF POLYSTYRENE

Rubber-modified impact grades generally exhibit good strength properties.
Homopolymer polystyrene has excellent clarity. Impact grades range from translucent to opaque.
Homopolymer and impact grades have good resistance to many mineral oils, alkalies, salts, the lower alcohols, and aqueous solutions of these compounds.

DISADVANTAGES OF POLYSTYRENE

Offers poor barrier for moisture vapor transmission.
Is dissolved by many hydrocarbons, ketones, higher aliphatic esters, and essential oils. In some instances chemical attack can be reduced by releasing residual stresses through annealing.
Containers cannot be made routinely by extrusion–blow molding.

4.2.3 Polycarbonate

Among the first uses for polycarbonate (PC) in packaging was in baby bottles, where its sparkling clarity, resistance to heat, and light weight made it an ideal glass replacement. Newer applications include 5-gallon water bottles, returnable milk containers, and other largeware items.

The polycarbonates are made from bisphenol A and carbonic acid. The chemical and solvent resistance of PC is similar to that of polyvinyl chloride (PVC). Generally speaking, PC exhibits good resistance to water, diluted organic and inorganic acids, oxidizing and reducing agents, and neutral and acid salts. There is also good resistance to mineral, animal, and vegetable oils and fats, and aliphatic and cyclic hydrocarbon solvents. Polycarbonate is attacked by alkalies, amines, ketones, esters, and aromatic hydrocarbon solvents. It is dissolved by methylene chloride, ethylene dichloride, chloroform, cresol, dioxane, and pyridine.

Polycarbonate has oxygen, water vapor, and carbon dioxide permeation rates that are 69, 2.4, and 10 times greater, respectively, than those of PVC. These ratings can be misleading, however, since they were derived from tests from the American Society for Testing and Materials (ASTM) that were applied to films less than 5 mils thick. For instance, actual water permeation tests in blow-molded bottles show that PC exhibits five times the water permeation rate of PVC.

Polycarbonate has a lower specific gravity (1.2) than PVC (1.315). This means that the gram weight of PC bottles can be 9% lighter than PVC bottles and still achieve the same wall thickness.

The heat deflection temperature of PC is very high. Tests by laboratories indicate that PC bottles can withstand temperatures of 212°F (boiling water temperature) without deformation. Polycarbonate is among the toughest materials in the thermoplastic resin family. Polycarbonate bottles fall just short of being unbreakable.

ADVANTAGES OF POLYCARBONATE

Good toughness, optical clarity, and gloss, as well as creep resistance and heat deflection qualities Light in weight, yet good tensile and flexural strength.

DISADVANTAGES OF POLYCARBONATE

Oxygen, carbon dioxide, and moisture barrier properties not as good as those of nitrile or PVC
Relatively high cost
Relatively difficult processing

4.2.4 "Barrier" Materials

Generally, all plastic containers offer some barrier to environmental conditions. Bottles made from polyvinyl chloride, nitrites, and polyesters, however, offer more across-the-board resistance to oxygen, carbon dioxide, and moisture than those made from other resins.

Polyvinylchloride. For many years PVC has enjoyed status as a superior packaging material for a variety of applications. Despite adverse publicity and the possibility of FDA restrictions on certain applications for PVC bottles, U.S. consumption has held steady, and strong future growth is anticipated. The basic component of a rigid PVC blow-molding compound is vinyl chloride monomer. Commercial production of vinyl chloride monomer starts with either acetylene or ethylene. Compounds for rigid PVC bottles consist of a mixture of as many as 15 or as few as 6 components. A typical compound consists of the following:

Ingredients	Parts by weight
PVC base resin	100.00
Impact modifiers	12.00
Processing aids	3.00
Lubricants	1.50
Stabilizers	3.00
Toners	0.05

ADVANTAGES OF PVC

Excellent rigidity

Better oxygen blocking (15–20 times) than polyethylene

Good barrier for aliphatic hydrocarbon solvents and dilute ester flavor ingredients

Better moisture barrier than nitrites.

Lower price per pound than nitrites but somewhat offset by lightweight nitrile

Excellent clarity and gloss

DISADVANTAGES OF PVC

Impact strength, generally fair at room temperature compared with polyethylene, is improving with development of new grades, and through orientation.

Moisture vapor barrier properties are one-fifth to one-tenth those of polyethylene.

Maximum hot-fill temperature is 150–160°F.

Inertness is far worse than polyethylene, and PVC is attacked by aromatic and chlorinated hydrocarbon solvents, concentrated esters, acetates, and ketones.

4.3 Polyester

The major commercial application using oriented polyester is bottles for carbonated beverages. Wide applications also appear feasible in the food and beverage, toiletries, and cosmetics, medicinal and health, and household chemical markets.

Polyesters are being developed for injection–blow molding and blow-molding use. Polyethylene terephthalate (PET) is derived from dihydric alcohol and dicarboxylic acid. From these basic chemicals come ethylene glycol and terephthalic acid. Through polymerization by condensation, a saturated polyester is produced known as PET for injection–blow molding only. Unsaturated polyesters have the capability to cross-link with other monomers (such as hexene) to produce a PET copolymer that can be blow-molded.

ADVANTAGES OF POLYESTER

Impact strength of oriented PET is excellent.

PET has excellent clarity.

PET has fine tensile and flexural strength that approaches the polycarbonates.

Compared with nitrile, polyesters have better clarity, toughness, and stress and crack resistance, as well as lower material costs and better moisture barrier properties.

DISADVANTAGES OF POLYESTER

PET's ability to resist oils, chemicals, or solvents is not quite as good as that of polyvinyl acetate (but better than nitrile), and it is attacked by strong acids, alkalies, and chlorinated hydrocarbons.

Its maximum product filling temperature is 160–165°F.

Food-grade PET requires special bottle manufacturing equipment. This equipment cannot produce handleware.

5 CONCLUSION

Packaging plays a key role in supporting the multifunctional nature of a product. From a marketing perspective packaging is important because of the message it conveys to the consumer on the shelf. Packaging is important to the product development staff because of the functional advantages it offers in terms of either improved stability or easier dispensing. In fact, some multifunctional products simply could not exist without the proper packaging. For these reasons and many others, the entire product development team can benefit by considering packaging design factors early in the new-product process.

BIBLIOGRAPHY

Erickson G. Shelf Presence. Monthly newsletter.
Hine T. The Total Package. Boston: Little, Brown, 1995.
Sorz, Bardocz, Radnoti. Plastic Molds and Dies. New York: Van Nostrand Reinhold, 1981.

13

Consumer Research
and Concept Development
for Multifunctional Products

Shira P. White
The SPWI Group, New York, New York, U.S.A.

There is a major shift in marketing that is especially important for multifunctional products (MFPs): customer focus vs product focus. A growing demand for customization and personalization is driving the development of new kinds of MFP and requires new kinds of customer information. It means that consumer research is more important than ever, and it calls for new methodologies to capture and use new kinds of data.

While the personal care industry has long known the importance of considering change in consumer demographics, multifunctional products present new challenges as demographics correlate to preferences for functional bundles. For example, a 50-year-old African-American woman is not going to care as much about sunscreen function, but may care more about exfoliation. She may prefer a different fragrance set than a 20-year-old woman. The number of preference choices multiply as the number of combined functions increases.

Development of successful MFPs is less likely to be related to the coincidental development of new technology and more likely to be the deliberate application of creative resources to market and technology research.

We know MFPs deliver more for consumers, whether they integrate multiple functions or have multiple uses. They are designed to serve more than one consumer need concurrently. We know they can, ideally, offer important benefits to consumers beyond what monofunctional products can offer, such as saving more time, space, and money. We also know MFPs are more complex than monofunctional products. This can make them harder to design or formulate, use, or maintain. This complexity is an important issue to explore with consumers.

On one hand MFPs can serve to expand your target market by appealing to a broader base of people, some of whom are attracted by one function, some of whom are attracted by other functions, and some who value the combination. Therefore, consumer research needs to cast a wider net.

On the other hand, MFPs can narrow a market by appealing only to people who prefer the combination of functions offered. Some people may prefer different combinations. Others, who do not think they need the whole combination every time, may prefer unbundled functions across multiple products. Some may believe they can get better quality in individual products or that buying individual products allows them more control. Therefore, consumer research needs to dig more deeply to better understand consumer need and preference.

1 CHALLENGES WITH MULTIFUNCTIONAL PRODUCTS

Multifunctional products present different kinds and different levels of challenges. Each challenge should trigger a new set of questions in market research.

1.1 It Can Be Difficult to Know the Best Mix of Functions and Features for Each Target Market

Positioning any product has challenges. But, with MFPs the challenges are in multiples. Marketers have to decide, often out of a large pot of possibilities, which functions to bundle and which features to promote. For example, consumers have different feelings about the fragrance in hair and skin products. These preferences can vary by culture and by social group. For instance, U.S. consumers tend to prefer a relatively light fragrance that dissipates quickly. Asian consumers tend to prefer a heavier scent that remains until the next use. Cleansing, whitening, conditioning, and other functions can evoke different sets of preferences. Researchers need to look at how functional bundle preferences vary by segment and subsegment, including cultural differences.

Although not usually considered as such, fragrance is a functional ingredient, with its own set of challenges. As functions are bundled in personal care products, fragrancing can present a few technical problems. The fragrance needs to be finely balanced to support the product's multiple roles. Marketers should explore fragrance preferences and perceptions related to each function as well as to the bundle. One important trend we observe is that customers are demanding enhanced performance and added functional benefits from the product's fragrance component. Marketers need to understand changing consumer preferences and expectations with respect to specific functions such as fragrance.

1.2 Determining the Optimal Number of Multifunction Combinations to Market Can Be Challenging

Diversifying the functional bundles and forms can also help companies spread the risks involved in developing a new product line. Conversely, flooding the market with too many similar products can hurt the whole line. To add to the quandary, the trend toward customization is increasing demand for more, and potentially, unlimited variations. Researchers need to assess the level of demand for variation as well as the nature of the variation in demand.

1.3 MFP Pricing and Positioning in the Marketplace Can Be Difficult

Nutriceutical and cosmeceutical ingredient suppliers see multifunctional products as an opportunity to leverage their technologies and expand their markets. Consumer products companies see them as an opportunity to increase both sales and margins. Multifunctional products can yield higher margins because they can command a higher price, sometimes five or six times as much as monofunctional competitors. But, the high price may not be worth the multifunctional benefit. Much of it depends on how the products are positioned.

Without understanding the multiple intricacies of each target, it is easy to miss the mark. For example, Kellogg failed to fully understand important aspects of their target's multiple preferences in the functional foods category. After spending millions of dollars in development, they still could not figure out how to position their MFPs. Their new Ensemble functional food product was touted to be high in fiber, as if that was big news. But consumers have known about high-fiber products for a long time already—they were nonplussed. Campbell Soup faced a similar disaster with their poorly positioned Intelligent Quisine functional food line.

In the absolute, a set of functions and features may seem like a sure hit based on various of target market research data. For example, in the functional foods category, it would seem as though high-fiber and health-hyped foods would be sure winners among aging, more health-conscious consumers. However, the Ensemble and Intelligent Quisine products were doomed because of errors in positioning and pricing.

Johnson & Johnson also missed. They developed a butter substitute that also functioned to lower cholesterol. The functional benefits seemed clear. The target of health-conscious and older consumers seemed right on the mark. But the positioning and pricing tripped them up. They placed their product, Benecol, in the dairy case, near real butter and other monofunctional butter substitutes. Even though consumers told researchers that they greatly valued the cholesterol-reducing function, they were blown away by the dramatic price difference: $7.29 for 5.9

ounces vs under $2.00 a pound for other butter substitutes. After trying different store placements and positioning variations, J&J rethought their strategy and considered promoting Benecol to physicians instead. This target presented new problems. Physicians knew that the relative benefit offered by the product was small in comparison to patients' needs to reduce cholesterol. And, ironically, with the exception of a few additions, such as added sunscreen function, physicians frequently counsel their patients to use simpler, monofunctional products.

There is no question: MFPs are tricky to position and price. Getting price/value relationships right can be a challenge because some functions and features are valued differently among different targets. Marketers need new tools to help unravel the complexities of price/multiple-value relationships among different market segments.

1.4 Managing Consumers' Expectations Can Also Be Challenging

Sometimes promised results are so long in coming, or learning proper use is so time-consuming, that consumers give up. Products that take weeks or months to show their multifunctional benefits often are abandoned before the formulations have had a chance to achieve results. Countless bottles of skin care products rotate through consumers' cabinets as any subtle wrinkle or pore reduction goes unnoticed. People move on to the next possibility, hoping that it can work sooner, or even at all. Patience levels need to be queried in consumer research studies. Super-high-margin Rembrandt toothpaste succeeded in spite of itself because consumers perceived that, over time, it was working to whiten their teeth better than other toothpastes. Dentists, however, agreed that there was actually no superior benefit. Researchers need to determine the specifics about how the consumer thinks the MFP will perform, as well as to assess their levels of expectations.

As products become more complex, it becomes a greater challenge to assure customers that individual parts or ingredients are working well and do not interfere with each other. Again, perception counts. Consumers may be afraid that MFPs may function less efficiently than their monofunctional counterparts. They may be concerned about what might happen if one of the multiple functions fails while the others work. They may even believe, as in the case of two-in-one shampoo/conditioner products, that the multiple functions cancel each other out. Marketers need to understand these consumer concerns.

Many MFPs are introduced without an adequate explanation of how they work or why they are better than earlier products. Confused consumers hurt sales. It is essential that consumers have a good understanding of how the multiple functions work individually and in concert. Marketers need to find out the level of information consumers really want or need so that they can sufficiently communicate benefits both in advertising and on packaging.

Sometimes the optimal mix of functions and features does not fit with the consumers' perceptions of the brand. The brand may need to be redefined and rebuilt to accommodate these new MFPs. Image and design are, essentially, functions serving to enhance a customer's aesthetic experience and increase confidence. Consumer research should explore these matters as part of the function bundle to determine levels of influence and preference.

2 KEY POINTS OF INQUIRY

Once traditional market research questions have been asked and the basics have been established, the multifunctional product developer needs to dig deeper and ask: What are the unarticulated needs of the market? Is there a new need for synergy? What value might a new MFP offer? What value can be added by combining functions?

Just because a company has the technological capability to combine functions does not mean its MFP will fly. Benefits must be meaningful to create value. Otherwise, consumers may prefer to stick with more familiar products that may be less expensive, or easier to use.

Sometimes, when marketers get it right, just one added ingredient can start a market boom. For example, there has been significant growth in industries such as skin care products because, for example, interest in anti-aging and sun protection have driven the development of new products that incorporate alphahydroxy acids (AHAs) and sunscreens. In recent years, over a thousand new products are launched annually, more than twice as many as a decade ago. AHAs have been responsible for much of this impressive growth. Marketers need to learn more and manage data better to get to these sweet spots.

In addition, customer input is becoming more important than ever. Results of consumer research must be used to actually help shape and optimize the product, not just to elicit approval or rejection of decisions already made. Research needs to advance to uncover the many untapped and changing opportunities for new MFP development.

2.1 Companies Need to Find New Ways to Explore Opportunities

There are a lot of uncovered opportunities to develop new MFPs. Some are outside a company's view set. Some opportunities have been here all along without being discovered by anyone. Some are the result of change. Marketers need better ways to uncover and track trends in consumer and competitor profiles. They need to dig outside their own sandboxes, and they need better ways to do that.

MFPs usually use combinations of existing technologies targeting a combination of needs that are already known about. Marketers can improve their chances if they can learn more about newly emerging technologies and newly emerging needs that specifically impact the potential for multiple function. Some of these efforts can target the future. But there are also likely to be more opportunities for today. Companies need to find out about enabling technologies up and down their supply chains. They need to find out about technologies in other industries. And, they need to find out what consumers really need and how they really feel, beyond what they say, about proposed multifunctional solutions. All these quests can lead to new opportunities for multifunctional products.

New solutions tend to create new problems. New problems are new opportunities. MFPs themselves can trigger needs for new MFPs. For example, now antiaging products must become antiaging/restorative products. Continued interest in AHAs and demand for mildness are driving changes in formulations. Since AHAs chemically strip the skin, chemists have looked to add MPDiol glycol and propylene glycol, which can help reduce physical irritation by creating a smoother product.

Marketers need to find new ways to think about multiple product use. Consumers may use different multifunctional products in ways not expected by developers. The problems that consumers may be experiencing in use may not all come to light. And, even if there are no surprises now, the world is changing faster and faster—use can change as a result of these changes.

2.2 Companies Need New Ways to Detect Patterns and Find New Correlations

As the world changes, new patterns in a range of behaviors occur. Demographics change. Information changes. Fashion changes. Competitors change. Capabilities change. Lifestyles change. Interests change. Culture changes. Knowledge changes. These and other changing areas need to be continually explored, monitored, and tested.

Early, when change is nascent, and new data begin to show up, companies need to be able to see patterns faster than their competitors. We have access to more data now than anyone has ever had in the history of the world. Companies need to see whether data are beginning to relate to each other in any new way. They need better ways of making sense of it all. And, they need better ways to turn data into knowledge and knowledge into ideas.

2.3 Companies Need New Ways to Capture Customer Information Over the Life of the Customer

Consumer segmentation is dynamic. Demographic and lifestyle changes can shift consumers from one segment to another. The customer–marketer relationship can be deepened and lengthened if these shifts and changing needs are anticipated, reducing customer acquisition costs, increasing revenues, and boosting profitability. Marketers need to study and respond to these changes with new product strategies, new functions, and new bundles.

3   NEW CONCEPT DEVELOPMENT
AND RESEARCH METHODOLOGIES

3.1   TrendScoping ⓈⓂ

Vitamins, AHAs, antibacterials, sunscreens, moisturizers, and gloss—they all grew out of consumer trends, and their various combinations grew out of the convergence of those trends. The earlier you can detect emerging trends and see their budding convergences, the greater your advantage.

One of the more common practices among market researchers is to focus on directly related trends, looking only at the perceived target market, the currently defined industry, and the most obvious pertinent issues. For example, a hair-coloring marketer would likely concentrate its trend research on women 35–65 years old, in a lower to midrange economic bracket, who have a fashion preference for "no gray," as well as technological developments in hair care and color science, and competitive home hair color marketers. We have found tremendous benefit in tracking a much wider variety of trends that can influence new product development, such as the following:

- Societal trends, beyond perceived target
- Demographic trends, beyond perceived target
- Lifestyle trends, beyond perceived target
- Fashion and design trends, beyond perceived target
- Related industry trends
- Parallel industry trends
- General trends outside the target industry
- Technology trends inside and outside the target industry
- Economic trends, beyond perceived target
- Political and regulatory trends

New ideas often come from the intersection of seemingly unrelated universes. By systematically conducting broader TrendScopes and considering a wider variety of potential convergences, marketers are more likely to discover new multifunctional opportunities ahead of their competition.

3.2   Exploratory Research

Well-rounded exploratory research initiatives can help greatly in detecting new patterns and correlations. Because MFPs are more complex, it is important to get information and input from a variety of sources, at a variety of levels, and at each phase of the product development process. The first phase is opportunity discovery and assessment. One very key source of inspiration and knowledge that is often overlooked is raw customer and expert input.

Before quantitative analyses are done, before strategies are fully set, before concepts are developed, it is extremely valuable to check out what a broad definition of current and potential stakeholders are doing, how they are feeling, what they are thinking, and where they are heading when they need to use the kinds of product that are relevant to your business. It is helpful, in particular, to explore their raw experiences. It is important, up front, to see potential opportunities through their eyes.

This kind of exploratory research can be done through both discussion and observation. There are a variety of interesting approaches.

One approach, developed by SPWI, is Rapid-Fire Exploration. We conduct a series of intense rapid-fire triads and/or one-on-one interviews with current and potential stakeholders. We probe broadly and quickly to elicit a range of gut insights and responses. We get an edge on emerging trends by working with "next-wave consumers" and "last-wave consumers," that is, people who will be entering and leaving the market within a few years. The determinants of next and last waves can be based on age, lifestyle, culture, and adoption profile, among other factors.

Another approach is observational. We can use a form of empathic or anthropological research, as described further later, to observe, on an exploratory basis, current and potential stakeholders in general settings. From these observations, we can learn what is important and what is changing with respect to what makes them tick. We explore their worlds. We scout out a useful range of emerging trends as a basis for further exploration. We look at whole systems to find causal relationships and gaps.

It is important to have an outside view in exploratory research. An unbiased, creative facilitator/observer can often probe more deeply and broadly than on in-house staffer, and may see unrecognized opportunities, pick up important signals and nuances, and elicit more objective information from the research participants.

3.3 Empathic Design Research Methodologies

Often the most important pieces of information for a product developer are the things people do not talk about, the things they cannot tell you when you ask, the things they may not even recognize themselves. The currently exalted "Voice Of the Customer" (VOC) is not enough. A deeper understanding of people is important in any new product development initiative. Given the complexities of MFPs, it is even more important to achieve, and sometimes more difficult. Marketers need to go beyond traditional research data to understand aspects of consumers' needs and desires that they are unable to articulate. Underlying meaning, context, drivers, systems, and influencers all need to be part of the research picture and they can include empathic methodologies.

Ethnography is the primary empathic methodology used in consumer research. With its roots in anthropology and sociology, it produces a detailed description of specific cultures as observed by researchers inside the subjects' environment. Progressive design and manufacturing firms have been using these methodologies, mainly over the past decade, but the practice has only recently begun to catch on with a few leading-edge consumer products companies.

Ethnography usually includes a blend of historical, observational, and interview methods. This typically works in an iterative process between observing and testing. However, some believe that empathic research should not include testing or even much interaction at all between the researcher and the subject.

Focus groups, interviews, and usability laboratories yield information from artificial contexts. Surveys yield numbers but no meaning. Empathic research gets to the real story underneath the staged probes and numbers. It produces information simply unobtainable through other research methodologies.

Empathic research is extremely valuable in getting to unarticulated and undiscovered needs. It is a means for discovery. By observing and interacting with real people in a variety of real contexts, researchers are able to see their product use and reactions to this use. Researchers can see how people have created their own alternative uses for products, and, potentially, their own product bundling efforts to achieve the benefits of multifunction. And, they find new ways of thinking and ask questions that they would not have even known to ask.

For example, alternative use can point to or trigger the need for multifunctional products. A study by the Food & Brand Lab at the University of Illinois found that 30% of respondents, motivated by convenience, have found new ways to use cleaning products, such as using laundry bleach to clean countertops; 28% of respondents, motivated by cost consciousness, use health and beauty items in different ways, such as Preparation-H to tighten facial pores and smooth out fine wrinkles; and 26% of respondents, motivated by health consciousness, use food in new ways, such as substituting yogurt for sour cream in a recipe.

Simply knowing about the trends in health, cost, and time consciousness would not likely yield insights to alternative or "underground" use. But observing people using products in their own natural environments, as they go about their daily life, can reveal these emerging opportunities as well as previously undetected problems. We find that it is extremely helpful to also observe patterns of use of related products, such as food products in a beauty products study.

Beyond numbers and verbal answers of traditional methodologies, empathic research works with visual information, creative interaction, multidisciplinary teams, objective facilitators.

Product developers may believe that they already know a lot about their category and about existing functionalities, or they may believe that they get the data they need from traditional qualitative and quantitative methodologies. That is true only with well-known products. With established products and functions, consumers are familiar enough to be able to articulate quite a bit about their needs and preferences. Rembrandt tooth-whitening bleach strips were relatively easy for consumers to envision because many were already familiar with tooth bleaching kits offered by their dentists. But, significantly, new concepts and the new bundling of functions create needs for different kinds of information.

Consumers think in terms of incremental differences: make it softer, cheaper, easier. But rarely are they able to think beyond their current circumstances to even imagine the possibility of a whole new solution. For example, consumers never asked for fax machines.

If a company has a new technology or a radically new concept, unlike any that consumers are currently familiar with, it is unlikely to elicit meaningful feedback. It is likely to produce confusion and rejection.

Watching consumers has always yielded obvious, but still tremendously valuable, basic information. Consider usability: Is the package difficult to open? Does the user have to resort to the manual, or are operating principles clearly telegraphed by the design? Are handles, knobs, and distances from the floor designed ergonomically? Does the user hesitate or seem confused at any point? What unspoken and possibly false assumptions are guiding the user's interaction with the product?

Traditional research tools unearth basic information about preference and ease of use. Empathic techniques find more, such as the following.

1. *Interactions with personal environments.*   Where do people use products? How do their environments affect product use? For example, with society becoming increasingly mobile, many women need to apply makeup on the run—in taxis, on trains and buses, in the bathroom at work, and, yes, even driving or walking down the street. To make the job easier and quicker, and the cosmetics themselves less bulky, some women began to use their blush both for cheeks and as eye shadow, or their lipstick both for their lips and as their blush.

2. *Personalization.*   How do people alter products to suit their own needs and preferences? What alternative uses have people discovered? What causes people to use what they use? What causes them to change? What functions or features have they bundled on their own? For example, some consumers discovered that they could use hair conditioner in place of a shaving cream for their legs because they usually did not have shaving cream—still a "men-thing"—around. We have not yet researched the catalysts and drivers that moved some consumers to use Preparation-H as a remedy for under-eye circles, but the story is sure to be interesting.

3. *Experience in use.*   How do people feel when they use products? For example, is the experience relaxing, pleasurable, frustrating, or nostalgic? What subtle aspects affect the users? For instance, how do they respond to fragrance, texture, or color? How do they react to compliments or other comments they receive from friends and family? Do they feel confident in its use? For example, the tingle in Noxzema Skin Cream told consumers that the product was working.

4. *Unarticulated problems.*   What problems do people encounter in using products? What problems do they encounter in daily life that might illuminate a

new product opportunity? What can they not do that they might want or need to do? For example, consumers know that their hair doesn't look the way it should a week after a salon visit, but they may not be able to articulate why. The development of new shampoo and conditioner products that "lock in" color to keep it from fading or turning, or even to boost color in between visits, was a successful solution to this unarticulated need.

Empathic Research uses a process that grows out of anthropology. It includes the following steps:

1. *Preparation.* An outside expert is chosen to help plan and facilitate the process. A team is formed, including representatives across functional areas such as marketing, R&D, consumer research, sales, and customer service. In some cases, it is helpful to invite range stakeholders from outside the company to join the team. It is important to include both outside, objective observers and development team members. Together, they determine the scope of interest, including definitions of the subject group, the observation team, and the environment to be observed. And they plan the field trips.

2. *Observation.* The key difference between this set of methodologies and others is that it is often more about watching than it is about questioning. The observers are generally "quiet." They may send out a few very broad, open-ended questions, and they will likely develop a list of more specific questions to be used later in the development process. The primary object of the observation is consumer experience. The experience of applying, wearing, and removing makeup, in a variety of conditions, is the key focus, not the makeup itself. As the process moves forward, researchers may interact more with their subjects to bring another dimension to the learning.

3. *Recording.* Because of the visual nature of this kind of research, it is usually best to videotape, photograph, and do an audio recording of the observations. It is important to be as unobtrusive as possible, to avoid disturbing or influencing the subjects in any way. These recordings capture much more than observers could with note taking. The visual references are often triggers for new ideas.

4. *Analysis.* As with the first parts of the process, it is critical to have a variety of minds interpreting the data. Different people see different things. Different experience bases offer different insights. Again, objectivity is important. The object of the analysis is to define a set of both current and potential problems and needs.

5. *Application.* In this step, the inside/outside team merges the data they gathered with the company's capabilities and goals. This is an extremely creative part of the process, in which product solution ideas are generated, then concepts are visualized and developed.

6. *Prototyping.* Prototypes are developed, whether they are conceptual prototypes, virtual prototypes, or physical prototypes, to test and refine the product concepts. In some cases, researchers introduce prototypes to consumers in

their own environments and start the observation process again. Sometimes we work with prototypes in User Development Groups℠, a methodology the SPWI Group developed, which combines elements of both qualitative research and creative development (see more on User Development Groups and more on prototyping further on in the chapter). We introduce the prototypes to groups of consumers/users and moderate specialized in-depth discussions, inviting the participants into the creative process. In addition to giving feedback, they actually join in to shape and improve the prototype. In the case of multifunctional products, prototyping can be a big help in optimizing the functional bundle, because it offers a more concrete base from which to work.

The output data include stories and anecdotes, visual vignettes, and snippets of new understanding. Cultural and behavioral themes emerge. The data pool keeps growing, and the team repeatedly dips in throughout the development process. New insights create new questions, which create new insights.

3.4   User Development and Expert Development

Qualitative and quantitative research techniques are used in asking questions and observing behavior. Regardless of the methodologies used, they have significant limitations. There is a real advantage to inviting users and experts into the creative development process, where they help to form new ideas and proactively shape concepts. SPWI designed a set of methodologies, known as User Development Groups℠ and Expert Development Groups℠, that leverages not only the knowledge, but also the creativity of users and experts.

3.4.1   User Development

It can be extremely useful to include a variety of user segments in the User Development Process. It's a good idea, for example, to work with a range of users from the most expert to the most novice. The experts will offer cutting-edge creative input, and the novices will offer unfettered, unjaded development contributions.

Lead Users.   Lead Users push the envelope. They know the latest news on products, technologies, and style. Whether they are individuals, groups, or companies, they spawn trends. They are the first on the block to play with hair color and sport orange hair (voluntarily), the first to fiddle with a computer to make it do a new thing, the first to ask for bleached teeth, the first with the hottest new car, or the first to self-tan. They are ahead of the market.

Lead Users will more easily understand new concepts, intricacies, and idiosyncrasies of the product category.

Many significant innovations can be attributed to lead users. Because they are out on the edge, Lead Users need things before everyone else does. Their new ideas come from pondering a problem or a potential solution, from playing around with components, from modifying and mixing to satisfy their own special requirements. Lead Users are the first to dream about multifunctionality and the first to try it.

Product developers can learn much from Lead Users, discovering ideas for new products and new improvements for existing products. Lead Users are an extremely valuable resource. In essence, they are developers themselves, and they far outnumber marketing and R&D executives.

Base Users. Base Users are typical customers. They range around the hump of the bell curve. They may or may not be relatively homogeneous—there can be multiple segments. They use products that have been well established by more advanced Lead Users. For example, they are the sea of glossy lips after the fashionistas have moved on to matte.

Potential Customers

VIRGINS AND NEOPHYTES.   These are potential customers, who can still be outside or just barely inside the target market. They can be too young. They can be uninitiated. They can be in a different economic bracket. They do not yet use anything in your category—For example, a 10-year-old girl not yet using makeup or a twenty-something with not even the slightest need for wrinkle reducers. What might they hope for or fantasize about? What are their impressions of current products and users?

COMPETITORS' CUSTOMERS.   Their hearts belong to someone else. For now.

Non-Users. These are people who do not use any products in your category, either as a matter of choice or because of lack of awareness—for instance, women who never go to the salon and men who never wear moisturizer; or manufacturers who never use silicone ingredients.

3.4.2   Expert Development

Experts can also be creative resources. On one hand, the more they know about something, the harder it may be for them to think of counterintuitive ideas. But, on the other hand, the more they know, the more paints they have in their paint box. Each new product development project can benefit from a carefully designed and tailored Expert Development Group℠. SPWI works with a select group from our Leading Edge Expert Network℠ to gain advanced insights as well as to create new concepts and concept components. Typical Expert Development Groups are intentionally diverse and customized to best serve the specific project. Representatives may include the following:

- **Industry and related experts,** such as cosmetics experts
- **Parallel industry experts,** such as fashion experts
- **Technology experts,** such as chemists or engineers
- **Social development experts,** such as psychologists or anthropologists
- **Cultural experts,** such as artists

3.5   Visual Techniques

3.5.1   The Zaltman Metaphor Elicitation Technique (ZMET)

The Zaltman Metaphor Elicitation Technique (ZMET) is a patented research tool, developed by Gerald Zaltman, Joseph C. Wilson Professor of Business Administration and a member of Harvard University's interdisciplinary initiative, "Mind, Brain, and Behavior." ZMET leverages knowledge from a wide variety of disciplines, including cognitive neuroscience, neurobiology, art and literary criticism, visual anthropology, visual sociology, semiotics, the philosophy of mind, art therapy, and psycholinguistics. Its principles have special relevance to the complex issues of multifunctional products. ZMET works with visual imagery. Its core premises are as follows:

- Most social communication is nonverbal.
- Thoughts occur as images.
- Metaphors are central to cognition.
- Cognition is grounded in embodied experience.
- Deep structures of thought can be accessed.
- Reason, emotion, and experience commingle.

ZMET is an interactive technique that uses an assortment of visual images collected by the research subjects themselves. The researchers guide the subjects through a series of probes and in-depth analytical conversations, based on the pictures. The images chosen by the subjects are metaphors for their thinking and they elicit deep, previously untapped thoughts and emotions. ZMET brings unarticulated needs to the surface of awareness, revealing new opportunities for product developers.

3.5.2   Visual Streaming℠

Visual Streaming is a technique developed by SPWI that is used both for research and for ideation. Like ZMET, Visual Streaming uses visual images as key tools. Subjects are shown a continuous stream of visual images in video, film, or slide format, and asked to respond to a series of questions as they watch. The visual images serve to trigger both unarticulated thoughts and new conceptual connections. Once the subjects have completed the series, a specially trained facilitator leads them in a discussion, seeking to clarify, qualify, expand, and flesh out their answers.

3.6   Prototyping the Market

The traditional progression, from concept to prototype to qualitative and quantitative research, to test marketing, has been transformed. High-tech consumer research techniques are now so sophisticated that test markets are no longer necessary. Products go straight from consumer research to national launch. We call it prototyping the market. The prototype becomes the product and the product becomes the prototype, live, in real time in the marketplace.

Microsoft was one of the first companies to prototype the market when they launched their notoriously buggy Windows Version 1.0. They were obsessed with speed, paranoid about competitive copycats, and frugal. Once they had sunk capital into product development they figured they might as well go to market to let customers buy it and try it. Essentially, Microsoft let the market do their beta testing, while generating revenue at the same time. Live prototyping can be a great way to let the market determine the optimal design, function and feature mix, communications strategy, positioning, and pricing of MFPs.

To avoid prohibitively high supermarket regional premiums, many marketers decided to forgo test marketing, take the plunge, and launch nationwide. Some multinationals use small European countries, such as Belgium, as their test markets. But, big country or small, marketers must become more experimental, adding or withdrawing new products across the board.

There are prototyping methods that can reduce risk before market launch. Marketing researchers can use three-dimensional models or samples in User Development Groups, where participants physically explore and modify the prototypes. Virtual reality prototyping can be used "virtually" the same way. For example, there are virtual reality applications that simulate supermarkets or other user experiences. These simulations make it possible to test multiple variations of a concept, as in concurrent engineering, allowing researchers to explore solution formulation, design, functional and feature bundles, without the time and expense of three-dimensional reality. Virtual reality research tools can save a company the tremendous cost of producing thousands of product samples for consumer testing. Some are advanced enough to allow the subject to move or rotate the product image as if they were really turning it over in their hand. As virtual reality technology advances, additional sensory simulations will be possible, such as virtual smell and feel.

3.7 Relationship-Based Research

Market research is moving increasingly online. It has revolutionized the way companies get their information, the way they market, and the way they relate to customers. Innovative data management technologies put that information to work, opening up new opportunities and building strong "personal" relationships with customers.

High-speed computing and data storage technologies now allow marketers to develop complex customer marketing databases. Some companies are able to collect, archive, cross-reference, and access a mind-boggling amount of data on specific customer needs, preferences, behaviors, issues, tendencies, and actual purchasing behavior. They then use sophisticated analytical techniques to turn this vast accumulation of data into actionable customer information. Marketers can cluster customer data by actual past behaviors as opposed to segmenting a small statistical sample.

There are multiple drivers of customer profitability. Multiple research techniques are needed to sort out the influences of each. A combination of statistical and financial analysis initiatives yields the most useful information. Marketers can combine a variety of traditional demographic and lifestyle segmentation techniques with purchasing data to create "transactional profiles." These profiles essentially enable segmentation by customer value. For example, a marketer can focus on high-value customers and, by cross-referencing innumerable data point combinations, can develop specific product strategies tailored for each attitude- or behavior-based subsegment. For instance, an affluent woman who prefers high-fashion glitz and an affluent woman who prefers conservative luxury can be motivated by entirely different things, even though they both bought the same lipstick.

To create transactional profiles, researchers first look at customers' purchasing behaviors over past years. They next look at their current characteristics in terms of lifestyle, life stage, and income, and then project potential scenarios of profitability in the future. Finally, they segment by profitability over time. By understanding how need and purchasing behavior patterns change, marketers can better understand how to stay on target with each profitability segment.

To best evaluate and target customer profitability segments, researchers should consider questions such as the following:

- How often and when does she buy related products?
- How much did the products cost?
- What and how much does she buy within the product category?
- How loyal is she? How long has she been a customer for a given set of products?
- Why and when does she move to the competition?
- What is her financial situation in terms of income, liquidity, security, and risk?
- How does she respond to different marketing and promotions tactics?
- How does all this change over time?

This new way to segment the market is exposing opportunities for new multifunctional product ideas. Companies can develop extremely targeted products, optimizing multifunctional bundles, positioning, and pricing. They can also support these products with equally targeted marketing and promotions strategies. Transactional profiling is proving to be a successful methodology, showing that it can yield a significantly improved customer response, more incremental revenue, and increased profitability.

Finally, the personal care industry can get really, really personal, as can any company now, in any industry. Internet and other new data management technologies are so advanced that they allow marketers to acquire, analyze, and organize an astounding amount of personal information from each customer to create a niche segment of "one." Each data-rich personal dossier enables marketers to customize the functions, forms, and features of their products for each individual consumer, "one-to-one."

One-to-One marketing helps by growing relationships with customers, one at a time. Sophisticated interactive websites, combined with new, highly adaptable design, manufacturing, and delivery technologies, are what make this incredibly personal connection possible. The personalized aspect of this kind of research can be advantageous for MFP development because it can deal so well with multiple scenarios, to mix and match super-quickly and effectively.

Traditionally, the marketer has been the aggregator of functions and features, selling integrated multifunctional products. With the level of customization that new technologies now deliver, customers can create their own personal mix of functions and features to form their own personal MFP. This means that the marketer is actually now unbundling functions and features and offering them in pieces, which has new implications for product formulations and design.

Customized MFPs need customized packaging, marketing, and communications. The universe of data collected, mined, and organized can help customize it all. For example, there can be 10 different communications strategies, based on the new, more finely sliced customer segmentation strategy. Now, with rich purchase behavior and preference information to beef up data profiles, the marketer can construct offers, communications, and even packaging templates with dozens of variable data fields in each.

The more personal a relationship is, the more carefully that relationship needs to be managed. Some companies use websites to probe and monitor customer activity. Some are interactive. Some maintain a 24/7 online dialogue with current and potential customers, often in real time, asking them questions and requesting feedback.

Customer Relationship Management (CRM) programs manage a steady inflow of customer information, which companies use to help keep their customers happy and loyal. CRM allows companies to quickly learn about changing needs and quickly develop new fitting solutions. Data management systems are so robust that they can set up an interactive information flow between every key department and each customer to dramatically improve product development initiatives. Beyond marketing, divisions such as R&D, sales, customer service, manufacturing, and even finance, can be in touch with a consumer, for an enterprise-wide relationship.

One example of a successful relationship-based MFP line is Procter & Gamble's reflect.com, sold exclusively online. P&G uses Internet-based research techniques via the reflect.com website to gather super-detailed personal information, from a variety of consumers, which may affect their cosmetics preferences and interests. P&G offers consumers the chance to create their own customized multifunctional or multifeatured cosmetics products.

Reflect.com is one of only about 50 online sites that offers customized products. Each customer can design her own combination of product functions and attributes. And, consumers have been jumping at the chance to craft the functional and feature bundles they want most. As of October 2000, reports showed that about 10% of the reflect.com site's 500,000 monthly visitors customized almost 50,000 combinations of products. About 20% were repeat purchases, and revenue has been increasing by over 50% each month.

P&G is attempting to build a relationship with each woman. They begin by asking each site visitor quite a few questions, creating an individual profile for each visitor. For example, a visitor interested in hair care will be asked to answer questions about her hair, product formulation, packaging preferences, and graphics. Every time the visitor returns to the site, she is asked additional personal questions, so that gradually and unobtrusively, P&G builds a rich bank of information that can be used to develop new and improved offerings. The profile can provide a better sense of the type of products and bundles in which each person may be interested, so the site can direct that person toward particular options and help her to make her choices.

With reflect.com, customers are able to communicate what kinds of products and what combinations they want, so they are really creating their own optimal multifunctional products. While still relatively small potatoes, online sales of high-end cosmetics are expected to rise from less than 1% of the $25 billion market in 2000 to 5% by 2005. Regardless of whether a manufacturer is interested in selling products online, the Internet is the unsurpassed tool for assessing multiple dimensions of consumer need and for gathering valuable information to help in multifunctional product development.

4 CONCLUSION

Consumers are getting more and more sophisticated. Technology is becoming more and more sophisticated. And, products are becoming more and more sophisticated. Sometimes it is hard to tell which came first, as with the chicken and the egg. But one thing is clear: consumer research techniques need to expand in scope to uncover new drivers, needs, and preferences—even more so with multifunctional product research.

Power is shifting to the customer, and so the marketer's focus must follow. But, listening to the Voice Of the Customer is not enough—it will yield only incremental gains. By using TrendScoping, as well as exploratory and empathic research techniques, marketers can learn more about the current and potential unarticulated needs of consumers and can tailor their multifunctional product offerings accordingly. With User and Expert Development Groups, marketers can leverage the creativity of customers and cognoscenti on the edge—they can become creative partners.

The market can become a massive beta test. By prototyping the market—introducing works-in-process products into the full marketplace, as opposed to a limited test market—marketers gain the advantages of being the first/early mover; they get data based on actual reality, as opposed to simulation or sampling; and they significantly reduce research costs.

As customers become more important and more demanding, marketers are seeking to build stronger relationships with them. The technology of the Internet, in particular, is helping marketers to get to know consumers better, enabling them to develop deeper, smarter relationships with individual customers. Marketers can gather and slice up new piles of data to segment more meaningfully. Those who segment by transactional profile, concentrate research on the whole life of a customer relationship, and continually develop new multifunctional products to fit her changing needs, will increase profits and reduce customer acquisition costs.

Marketers now have the ability to research, develop, communicate, and sell on a personal, one-to-one basis, taking the axiom "It's not just what you know, but who you know," to a whole new level of meaning. Product developers have an unprecedented opportunity to meet personal needs and preferences even more with multifunctional products by enabling consumers to help design the functional and feature bundles that suit them best. And, multifunctional product marketers can now use the new scope and power of consumer research and Customer Relationship Management programs to build healthy, profitable relationships with customers on a long-term basis. If marketers can raise the level of creativity in ideation and concept development to at least the same levels of quality, it will be a multifunctional "slam dunk."

Chapter was written by Shira P. White, president and CEO of SPWI, a leading consulting firm specializing in innovation management and new product development. Inquiries and comments are welcome. SPWI, 189 West 89th Street, Suite 11C, New York, NY 10024. 212-706-0242. wwwow@earthlink.net

BIBLIOGRAPHY

RJ Babyak. Marketing with a vision: Multigenerational product development at GE Appliances. Appl Manuf 43(7), July 1995.

J Beerling. Formulating and fragrancing multi-functional shampoos. Manuf Chem 64(11):18, November 1993.

J Beerling. Towards multi-functional shampoos. Drug Cosmet Ind 154(4):30, April 1994.

D Burman. The design to cost (DTC) approach to product development. Trans AACE Int, V11–V13, 1998.

JD Cook, P Georgiadis. Packaged goods: It's time to focus on product development. McKinsey Qu No. 2:91, March 22, 1997.

TC Cook. Steps to new product market success: Packaging by the numbers. Packaging 38(4):11, March 31, 1993.

L de Chernatony, PJ Rosenberger III. Virtual reality techniques in NPD research. J Market Res Soc 37(4):345, October 1995.

D Fost. Improving on nature: Enhancing functionality in the search for the ideal ingredient. Drug Cosmet Ind, 159(4):46, October 1996.

I Greig. Facing brand changes. Marketing, p 17, August 22, 1991.

S King. Market research firm turns to computers to test new ideas. Kansas City Bus J 15(39):11, June 13, 1997.

D Leonard, JF Rayport. Spark innovation through empathic design. Harvard Bus Rev, p 102, November/December 1997.

L Light, R Furchgott. If you like the suit, click here. Bus Week, p 8, November 17, 1997.

LM Lodish, DJ Reibstein. New gold mines and minefields in market research. Harvard Bus Rev, p 168, January/February 1986.

DJ Morrow. A medicine chest or a grocery shelf? New York Times, Section 3, page 1, column 1, December 12, 1999.

I Nonaka, H Takeuchi. The new new product development game. Harvard Bus Rev, p 137, January/February 1986.

RJ Ortt, JPL Schoormans. Consumer research in the development process of a major innovation. J Market Res Soc, 35(4):375, October 1993.

B Perry. Seeing your customers in a whole new light. J Qual Participation 21(6):38–41, November/December 1998.

DH Pink. Metaphor marketing. Fast Company, pp 214–230, April/May 1998.

L Platts. A new method for consumer testing fragrances. Soap Perfum Cosmet 63(10):53, October 1990.

M Rogers. Mirror says: reflect.com among the fairest of them all. Inside 1 to 1, October 5, 2000.

M Sonnack. Creating breakthroughs at 3M. Harvard Bus Rev, p 47, September/October 1999.

R Snowdon. Why JWT is now asking the obvious. J. Walter Thompson Co, Analysis. Marketing, p 16, September 14, 1995.

T Stevens. From concept to customer. Ind Week, p 31, September 21, 1998.

SG Thomas. Getting to know you.com. U.S. News & World Rep. pp 102–112, November 15, 1999.

M Van Clieaf. Identifying your most profitable customers. Bus Q 61(2):54, December 1996.

Why new products are bypassing the market test. Manage Today, p 12, October 1995.

J Wilck. Baby boomers and natural ingredients lift personal care. Chem Market Rep 251(19):SR3, May 12, 1997.

G Zaltman. Rethinking market research: Putting people back in. J Market Res XXXIV:424, Fall 1997.

Index